The Essential MD-PhD Guide

The Essential MD-PhD Guide

Mark J. Eisenberg, MD, MPH
Director, MD PhD Program
Director, Cardiovascular Health Services Research Program
McGill University
Montréal, Quebec

Andrea L. Cox, MD, PhD
Director, MD PhD Program
Johns Hopkins University
Baltimore, Maryland

Mc Graw Hill

New York   Chicago   San Francisco   Athens   London   Madrid   Mexico City
Milan   New Delhi   Singapore   Sydney   Toronto

The Essential MD-PhD Guide

Copyright © 2021 by McGraw Hill. All rights reserved. Printed in the United States of America. Except as permitted under the United States Copyright Act of 1976, no part of this publication may be reproduced or distributed in any form or by any means, or stored in a data base or retrieval system, without the prior written permission of the publisher.

1 2 3 4 5 6 7 8 9 LCR 26 25 24 23 22 21

ISBN 978-1-26046227-2
MHID 1-260-46227-7

The editors were Karen Edmonson and Christina M. Thomas.
The production supervisor was Catherine Saggese.
The text designer was Mary McKeon.
Project management was provided by Garima Poddar, KnowledgeWorks Global Ltd.

Cataloging-in-publication data for this book is on file at the Library of Congress.

McGraw Hill books are available at special quantity discounts to use as premiums and sales promotions, or for use in corporate training programs. To contact a representative please visit the Contact Us pages at www.mhprofessional.com.

CONTENTS

Preface

The *Essential MD-PhD Guide* is an all-inclusive guide to the MD-PhD pathway. The book is a collaborative effort between MD-PhD students at McGill University in Montréal, Québec and Johns Hopkins University in Baltimore, Maryland. The purpose of the *Essential MD-PhD Guide* is to give an in-depth overview of the MD-PhD pathway—an intensive program of study leading to both MD and PhD degrees—with the ultimate goal of producing exceptional physician scientists who will make meaningful contributions to the medical field.

More than 130 MD-PhD programs are offered in North America. These programs allow students to graduate with both MD and PhD degrees following approximately eight years of medical and graduate studies. MD-PhD programs are intended to produce highly motivated and well-trained graduates who will establish themselves as leading physician scientists in a whole range of scientific and clinical domains. Graduates have the challenging yet rewarding task of identifying research questions at the bedside, studying these questions in the laboratory, and bringing novel therapies back to the patients who need them.

Upon completing their training, MD-PhD graduates often pursue careers at academic medical centers where they provide patient care and lead research laboratories, but many physician-scientist careers are available and provide the opportunity for those who understand patient care and research to make discoveries. Graduates are represented in any clinical domain ranging from primary care and internal medicine specialties to surgical subspecialties, public health, and many more. Similarly, graduates can be found in any research domain ranging from genetics, to epidemiology and health services research, to immunology, oncology—with too many to name! While their clinical and research domains may vary, what MD-PhD graduates have in common is their love of and commitment to both high-quality patient care and innovative medical research.

The *Essential MD-PhD Guide* provides a thorough overview of the issues facing MD-PhD students throughout all parts of their training. Because each chapter is written by one or more students, a variety of perspectives are presented. Some issues are covered in more than one chapter, allowing for viewpoints from Canadian and US perspectives, viewpoints from trainees of diverse backgrounds, as well as viewpoints from students and graduates in various stages of their careers (medical school, graduate school, residency, fellowship, and faculty). Each chapter begins with a short description of what stage the students were in at the time that the chapter was written. In addition, we begin each chapter with five key take-home messages that are addressed in detail in the ensuing chapter.

The *Essential MD-PhD Guide* is a must-read book for those considering careers as physician-scientists as well as for students currently enrolled in MD-PhD programs. The book provides a comprehensive review that will allow students to get the most out of their search for and time in an MD-PhD program and which will allow them to position themselves to have successful careers as physician-scientists. The Guide is filled with first-hand experiences and practical advice. It leads the readers through topics such as choosing a program, navigating the early years of medical school, selecting a research laboratory and project, and negotiating the transitions between medicine and research and back again. The Guide also provides advice on choosing clinical rotations, residency programs, and fellowships, as well as the pursuit of different career options for MD-PhD graduates.

As directors of the MD-PhD programs at McGill and Johns Hopkins, it has been our pleasure to work on this collaborative effort. In addition to all the MD-PhD students and graduates who have authored or coauthored chapters, we are indebted to a variety of individuals without whom this book would not have come to fruition. We would first like to thank Matthew Dankner for skillfully leading the early stages of planning and content development. We would particularly like to thank Amir Razaghizad for managing this project. It required coordination of a large number of authors and reviewers. Amir expertly shepherded all the many drafts and revisions to a successful conclusion. We are indebted to our student reviewers including Etienne Maes, Jessica Petricca, Joan Miguel Romero, Judy Chen, Mark Sorin, Matthew Hintermayer, Michael Luo, Owen Chen, Sarah Lepine, Sarah Maritan, Scott Ehrenberg, and Tarek Taifour. We are also indebted to our faculty reviewers including Drs. David Buckeridge, Lysanne Campeau, Jenny Lin, Brent Richards, Jacquetta Trasler, and Pia Wintermark. Special thanks are owed to Dr. Yvonne Hung and Ben Wexler for editorial assistance. Finally, we would like to express our thanks to our families and colleagues for their encouragement and patience during the many months it took to prepare the *Essential MD-PhD Guide*.

Having careers in which we can provide patient care and conduct research is an honor and a privilege. Balancing what amounts to two separate careers can be challenging. Each requires specialized knowledge and a unique skillset. The MD-PhD career path is not for everyone. For those who decide to pursue this path, however, it is exceptionally rewarding and fulfilling. It is our hope that you will find the *Essential MD-PhD Guide* to be an indispensable guide that will help you in your own voyage of discovery.

Mark J. Eisenberg, MD, MPH   **Andrea L. Cox, MD PhD**

Introduction

The MD-PhD Roadmap
Written by Owen Chen, Sarah Maritan, and Joan Miguel Romero

Sarah Maritan is a first-year student in McGill University's MD-PhD program. She received her Bachelor of Science degree in Life Sciences, and her Master of Science degree in Pathology and Molecular Medicine, both from Queen's University in Kingston, Ontario. Her research focuses on the cellular signaling mechanisms regulating cancer progression, particularly the pathways underlying tumor cell movement and metastatic growth.

Joan Miguel Romero is a first-year MD-PhD student at McGill University. He completed his Honors Bachelor of Science degree in Pathobiology and Immunology and his Master of Science degree in Laboratory Medicine and Pathobiology at the University of Toronto. His research is aimed at understanding the antitumor immune mechanisms involved in pancreatic cancer.

Owen Chen is a first-year MD-PhD student at McGill University. Prior to medical school, he completed both his Bachelor and Master of Science degrees in Biochemistry at McGill. He is currently pursuing his research at McGill's Goodman Cancer Research Centre, where he studies cell cycle dysregulation in cancer.

Introduction

This book aims to provide an overview of the process of becoming a physician scientist. In particular, it focuses on MD-PhD programs, which integrate components of research and medical doctorate training into a single program. As this book is intended for readers at all stages of training, we have divided this book into sections: (I) Applying for MD-PhD Training, (II) Early Days in Medical School, (III) The Transition to Graduate School, (IV) Transitioning Back to Medical School, and (V) Residency, Fellowship, and Your First Job. The book concludes with section (VI) Physician-Scientist Wellness, with chapters applicable throughout all aspects of training. Within each section are chapters related to that phase of the MD-PhD training pathway, including information on specific milestones, first-hand accounts of experiences in the phase, and suggestions to help you during your training.

As an MD-PhD training pathway can be complex, this section of the book will serve as a brief outline of the important steps. Below is a diagram representing the typical MD-PhD training pathway, particularly as it pertains to combined programs, with the afore-mentioned sections numbered in the figure. This schematic is followed by an explanation of the pathway, with references to specific book chapters in parentheses that you can use to guide your reading.

The MD-PhD Roadmap:

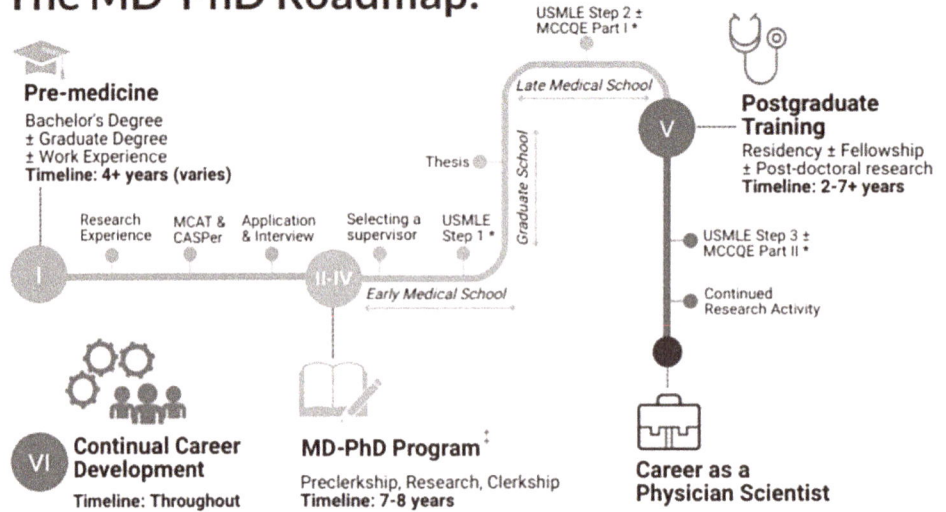

USMLE Step 2 ±
MCCQE Part I *

Late Medical School

Pre-medicine
Bachelor's Degree
± Graduate Degree
± Work Experience
Timeline: 4+ years (varies)

Thesis

Graduate School

Postgraduate Training
Residency ± Fellowship
± Post-doctoral research
Timeline: 2-7+ years

Research Experience

MCAT & CASPer

Application & Interview

Selecting a supervisor

USMLE Step 1 *

USMLE Step 3 ±
MCCQE Part II *

Continued Research Activity

I

II-IV   Early Medical School

V

Continual Career Development
Timeline: Throughout

MD-PhD Program ‡
Preclerkship, Research, Clerkship
Timeline: 7-8 years

VI

Career as a Physician Scientist

‡ Program structure may vary.
* USMLE and MCCQE are the licensing examinations for the United States and Canada, respectively.

Section I: Applying for MD-PhD Training

Prior to applying to an MD-PhD program, it is important to determine the suitability of this training pathway (Chap. 1), and consider which programs are best suited for the prospective applicant based on their goals and circumstances (Chap. 2). The MD-PhD pathway starts very similarly to the path of a pre-med student seeking admission to medical school; MD-PhD applicants have completed or are in the process of completing an undergraduate program, they may have completed a post-undergraduate program (a master's degree for example), or they may be currently working. One distinction between an MD-PhD applicant and an applicant to a regular medical program is that the MD-PhD applicant should have substantial research experience prior to applying to medical school. This experience is paramount to a strong application (Chap. 3), demonstrating interest in both medicine and research. Aside from this, MD-PhD applicants then go through the same application process as applicants for the regular MD program. This involves keeping up with extracurricular activities and research, taking the Medical College Admission Test (MCAT, Chap. 4) and the Computer-Based Assessment for Sampling Personal Characteristics (CASPer, Chap. 5) (if applicable), completing online applications, and if invited, attending interviews (Chap. 7). MD-PhD applicants will often have to complete supplemental applications, obtain letters of reference specific to their research experiences (Chap. 6), and attend separate PhD interviews in addition to interviews required for the MD portion (Chap. 7).

Section II: Early Days in Medical School

Once matriculated, most MD-PhD students begin an approximately eight-year journey, completing both undergraduate medical education and graduate studies. The layout of MD-PhD programs varies between medical schools. Many MD-PhD students follow a modified timeline that integrates their medical education with their research (Chap. 8). The typical format of an MD-PhD program is as follows: pre-clerkship, graduate studies, and clerkship. Most MD-PhD students start their programs as medical students learning the basic science of medicine in the classroom—these are the pre-clerkship years, which last around two years, or roughly the first half of medical school. For American and Canadian students who want to pursue residency and/or fellowship in the United States, this is the time to prepare for the United States Medical Licensing Examination (USMLE) Step 1 (Chap. 21), which is usually taken at the end of the second year. After pre-clerkship, MD-PhD students at most schools transition into their PhD programs for approximately three to four years, which can be preceded by a research rotation in some institutions (Chap. 9) to help select a supervisor (Chap. 10).

Section III: The Transition to Graduate School

Early in their graduate studies or possibly before formally beginning their PhD, students may begin discussing different thesis project ideas with their supervisors (Chap. 11). In addition to their research, students take graduate level courses and complete any required qualifying exams. An important component of graduate studies involves demonstrating strong research productivity (Chap. 12), typically in the form of attending conferences, presenting research findings, and in particular, publishing research papers (Chap. 13). As an MD-PhD student, it is also important to maintain clinical knowledge and find ways to integrate and maintain what was learned in the first phase of medical school during PhD training (Chap. 14). The final component of the PhD degree involves the completion of the experimental work of the project (Chap. 15) and the writing (Chap. 16) and defense of the thesis. Other skills relevant to your development as a researcher and a physician, such as the ability to successfully network (Chap. 17), are also cultivated during your PhD training.

Section IV: Transitioning Back to Medical School

After completion of the PhD, students return to the MD stream for about two years. There are steps they can take to help prepare for the transition back into medical school (Chap. 18). During this last phase of training, students select rotations and electives (Chap. 19) in different medical and surgical specialties during clerkship, where they learn the clinical skills necessary to become residents. MD-PhD students are typically integrated with a new cohort for the remainder of their training, and with this comes the excitement of new knowledge and new colleagues (Chap. 20). During this stage of medical training, American medical students take Step 2 of the USMLE (Chap. 21). During the final year, students apply to residency programs and prepare for their interviews (Chap. 22). Students then match into a residency program, and graduation follows. Canadian students typically take the Medical Council of Canada Qualifying Examination (MCCQE) Part I after the fourth year of medical school (Chap. 21).

Section V: Residency, Fellowship, and Your First Job

Depending on the program, postgraduate medical training ranges from two to seven years, or even longer. This is a time of intense clinical training as residents are developing skills to become independent practicing physicians. The first year, intern year, can be particularly intimidating, but provides an important foundation for your continued training (Chap. 23). During this transition, it is important to consider how to combine research with postgraduate medical training (Chap. 24). MD-PhD graduates may find themselves pursuing a residency program that has a significant portion of time dedicated to research, or in many cases, when protected research time is limited, they may choose to pursue research on their own time. Residents in the United States complete Step 3 of the USMLE during residency, whereas trainees in Canada take the MCCQE Part II (Chap. 21). MD-PhD graduates may pursue additional clinical training by completing fellowships and/or research training in postdoctoral programs (Chap. 25). These options entail an additional one to two years depending on the program and number of fellowships one wants to complete. Coming out of their residency or fellowship, MD-PhD graduates are well prepared to start an independent career as a physician-scientist (Chap. 26), with rewarding and diverse career options ahead of them (Chap. 27).

Section VI: Physician-Scientist Wellness

Several aspects of a physician-scientist training career path involve moments of stress and moments of elation, and it is important to acknowledge these times as one progresses through this unique career. There are many opportunities that do not fit exactly into the framework of the training pathway, but deserve to be addressed. Because of the long nature of this training pathway, some may encounter personal challenges and it is worth considering how to balance this with one's career (Chaps. 28 and 29). Hopeful and current students should be aware of how physician-scientists can best impact society (Chap. 30). Finally, the book acknowledges the need for a more diverse physician-scientist workforce and presents strategies for success in the face of systemic challenges for MD-PhD students from underrepresented populations (Chap. 31).

Conclusion

In this section, we have provided a brief overview of the MD-PhD pathway. By summarizing the sections and referencing the respective chapters, we hope this will facilitate the reading of this book. The journey to completing medical school and a PhD requires careful planning, patience, persistence, and hard work. You will come across many hurdles along the way, but this education and career pathway is a rewarding one.

PART I

Applying for MD-PhD Training

1

Is the MD-PhD Path Right for You?

Matthew Dankner

Matthew Dankner *is a fifth-year MD-PhD student at McGill University. He is a Montreal native who graduated from McGill University with an honours bachelor of science in Anatomy & Cell Biology before joining the MD-PhD program. For his PhD studies, Matthew is involved in basic, translational, and clinical research in the area of metastatic brain tumors.*

INTRODUCTION

If you're reading this book, you've probably at least entertained the possibility of enrolling in a combined MD-PhD program. Before you apply to one of these programs, there are a number of important questions you must ask yourself. Make sure to answer honestly. MD-PhD training can be the start of a wonderful and rewarding career trajectory, but it is a long and rigorous program. You must be truly committed to gain acceptance to such a program, to thrive there once admitted, and to continue thriving later in your career. This chapter will serve as a decision guide for potential applicants, helping them understand what an MD-PhD entails and whether it is right for them.

WHAT IS AN MD-PhD PROGRAM?

MD-PhD programs are intensive programs that simultaneously train students to become proficient in medicine and research. These programs exist as a part of the effort to develop the next generation of physician-scientists.

WHAT YOU NEED TO KNOW

- Physician-scientists are medical doctors who spend a significant proportion of their time doing research.
- MD-PhD programs are specifically designed for students who want to have careers that combine medicine with research.
- MD-PhD programs integrate medical school with a research-based PhD. Other pathways exist to becoming an MD-PhD physician-scientist, including doing a PhD before medical school or as a part of postgraduate residency or fellowship training.
- MD-PhD program graduates are uniquely positioned to impact biomedical research.
- Given the long duration of training, potential applicants to MD-PhD programs must seriously consider whether this is the right career path for them.

WHAT IS A PHYSICIAN-SCIENTIST?

Physician-scientists are invaluable for the medical community, as they act as a bridge between the worlds of clinical medicine and research. They are defined as medical doctors who spend a significant proportion of their time doing research, while still caring for patients or performing clinical duties. This allows them to identify and understand the pressing clinical needs that require thorough investigation through research. For most physician-scientists, at least half of their time is spent conducting research. Substantial medical improvements are made thanks to physician-scientists, even though they make up a small minority of all medical doctors and an even smaller percentage of scientists.

WHAT DIFFERENT PATHS EXIST FOR MD-PhD PROGRAMS?

Multiple structures for MD-PhD programs exist in North America. However, they uniformly integrate medical and PhD studies, with students following an unconventional path in both medical and graduate school. In the most commonly applied program structure, students begin with the classroom phase of medical school (1–2 years), followed by their entire PhD research (typically 3–4 years), before returning to medical school to complete their clinical clerkship. The typical MD-PhD program takes 7–9 years to complete, with 4 years of medical school and the remainder in graduate school; each university has its own time-to-completion standards for MD-PhD students.

WHAT AREAS OF RESEARCH DO MD-PhD STUDENTS AND PHYSICIAN-SCIENTISTS WORK IN?

The majority of MD-PhD students perform laboratory research. This can come in the form of fundamental or translational research. Fundamental research or "basic science" aims to understand the molecular underpinnings of disease entities or other health-related phenomena. Many MD-PhD students choose to focus their research in this area in order to learn the skills needed to think about abstract research questions and design and perform experiments to address them. Meanwhile, translational research uses wet-lab techniques and/or epidemiological approaches to directly address patient-centered research questions in attempts to improve patient care by going beyond the wet lab and into the clinic. MD-PhD trained physician-scientists are optimally equipped to make important strides in this area of research colloquially referred to as bench-to-bedside research.

While not an absolute rule, MD-PhD students tend to perform their PhD research in areas related to human health. Students working in virtually any field of science can conduct research with direct applications to health care, for example, physics (nuclear medicine, radiology) or chemistry (drug design/development). In addition to the above laboratory-based PhDs, MD-PhD students can also work in epidemiology to study health and disease at the population level, or study social sciences and economics to better understand societal determinants and other factors important in human health. It is evident that nearly any area of research can fit with an MD-PhD. For this reason, no interested student should shy away from an MD-PhD program thinking that their area of expertise cannot be tied to their clinical career in some way.

WHAT HAPPENS AFTER THE MD-PhD DEGREE IS COMPLETED?

Because MD-PhD students are trained with the intention of becoming physician-scientists at academic institutions, they often undergo further specialized medical training after graduation. This normally is broken down into a residency that can take anywhere from 2 years for family medicine to 5 or more years for internal medicine or surgical subspecialties (with variation between locations, specialties, etc.). This is often followed by a clinical or postdoctoral fellowship that can involve further clinical training, research training, or both. After all this training, one can finally begin working in a faculty position as a physician-scientist. Normally, MD-PhDs will be hired as physician-scientists, but they can also become full-time physicians, full-time researchers, or engage in a number of alternate career trajectories, such as industry, media, or politics. In almost all cases, MD-PhD graduates use knowledge and insights gained from both their clinical and research training in their careers. It is important to emphasize that physician-scientists can practice in any specialty or subspecialty of medicine to complement their research career.

Following the most common trajectory, working as a physician-scientist is a varied, intellectually stimulating, and challenging career. A physician-scientist spends at least half of their time doing research, with the remainder spent in clinical practice. Many physician-scientists spend up to 75% of their time on research.

WHAT SHORT-TERM INCENTIVES ARE THERE TO COMPLETE AN MD-PhD PROGRAM?

There are a number of short-term incentives to joining an MD-PhD program. First, for someone who wants to become a physician-scientist, the MD-PhD program offers the opportunity to be fully immersed in uninterrupted research without clinical or other life responsibilities that usually emerge later on in residency (e.g., having children). Fortunately, the majority of MD-PhD programs provide funding to their students in the form of free tuition, a stipend, or both. This is in order to attract students, given the high cost of medical school and the opportunity cost of graduating later than those doing an MD degree. The funding schemes offered by MD-PhD programs vary widely and are further discussed later in this chapter. If you are a potential applicant considering applying to an MD-PhD program, reach out to current MD-PhD students or program graduates at your institution to ask them any pressing questions you may have and to get the perspective of someone on the physician-scientist career path.

ALTERNATIVES TO THE MD-PhD CAREER PATH

It is important to note that MD-PhD programs are not the only route to becoming a physician-scientist. MDs without PhD training can typically be physician-scientists if they undergo significant research training in their residency and/or fellowship. As an alternative to obtaining a PhD during medical school, many MD-PhDs get their PhD training during their residency or fellowship. An advantage to this trajectory is that the research will be closer to the field a trainee ultimately works in. However, it becomes difficult to take on focused research training at this stage because of a significant clinical workload and increased family obligations at this later stage of training for many individuals. This becomes particularly problematic for trainees pursuing wet-lab research. These alternative career paths to becoming a physician-scientist will be further discussed in Chapter 27.

WHAT DOES IT TAKE TO BE ACCEPTED TO AND SUCCEED IN AN MD-PhD PROGRAM?

Getting into an MD-PhD program is not easy, but it's certainly possible for keen and focused students. Those entering an MD-PhD program can have either a bachelor's or a master's as their most advanced degree. Some programs may allow junior PhD or first-year medical students to enroll, with the intention of taking a break from graduate school to begin medical school, only to return to the lab later on.

Academic background

MD-PhD programs are not reserved only for students who excelled in every class during their undergraduate degree and have a perfect MCAT score. Having good grades is extremely important, and the average grade point average of MD-PhD enrollees is typically higher than their MD counterparts. However, as in medical school admissions, there is room for students who have overcome adversity in their academic careers or life trajectory. Students from many different backgrounds can gain entry to an MD-PhD program. The most important criterion is being able to convincingly demonstrate one's potential of developing into a strong physician and researcher with a clear vision and understanding of the long path ahead.

While MD-PhD programs can be inclusive to all students, there are still important criteria that need to be fulfilled by any student joining such a program. Students must show a certain level of academic excellence that instills confidence that they will be able to complete both medical school and a PhD. In addition to academics, other activities needed for entrance to medical school are required for admission to an MD-PhD program. These include, but are not limited to, volunteering, experience in the health care system, and having unique and diverse life experiences. This is especially important to consider when deciding whether the MD-PhD path is right for you, because many programs mandate that students are first accepted into medical school before they are considered for admission to the combined MD-PhD program.

Research experience

In addition to the criteria for gaining admission to medical school, applicants to MD-PhD programs must also have substantial research experience and the drive not only to continue with research in the form of a PhD, but also to envision themselves as physician-scientists. Many MD-PhD programs require applicants to submit a document outlining their previous research experience and explaining their rationale for wanting to enroll in an MD-PhD program.

The research experience criteria for MD-PhD program admission can vary widely. As a general rule, more research experience is better, but applicants can be competitive with less experience if they have a clear vision in mind and can speak eloquently about their research. Publications are not necessary, given the fact that many applicants are current undergraduate students, but they do help in making an applicant stand out.

Interviews

After submitting their applications to an MD-PhD program, applicants who pass an initial evaluation (GPA, volunteering, research experience, etc.) are invited to an interview. Normally, separate interviews take place for the MD and the PhD portion of the program. While the medical school interview is usually the same as that being done by applicants to the MD program, the PhD portion of the interview is unique to MD-PhD applicants. The goal of this interview is to assess candidates' knowledge related to their research area of interest, their commitment to complete the program, and their level of interest in the program. As mentioned above, most programs require that students are first accepted into the MD portion before they can be considered for the MD-PhD program.

In terms of preparing for the MD-PhD–specific interview, there are a few important ways in which applicants can prepare. They should be able to fluently discuss their research experiences, provide an explanation for why they want to join the MD-PhD program, and show that they understand what the program entails, including the duration of training in this career path. This can be improved upon by practicing mock interviews with peers, research supervisors, or current MD-PhD students.

WHAT ARE THE ADVANTAGES OF DOING AN MD-PhD PROGRAM?

The benefits of doing an MD-PhD program are numerous. Most importantly, you have the opportunity to become an expert in both medicine and research. This makes for an extremely rewarding and versatile career where you can benefit your own patients, as well as many more patients in the future and around the globe, through your research. Since research training begins in the early phases of medical training, progress can be built upon while returning to medical school and residency. This contrasts with other physician-scientist career paths, where the main introductory exposure to high-level research occurs only near the end of training, leaving less time to fully develop skills before taking on a faculty position.

Being an MD-PhD student makes you stand out compared to other MDs and PhDs throughout your training and for the rest of your career. Of course, being enrolled in an MD-PhD program by no means assures your success in any particular area, but the prestige that comes with being an MD-PhD student will help in your future. Whether justified or not, professors and attending physicians will generally have greater faith in your ability to conduct and finish a research project if you are an MD-PhD student and will be more eager to invest their time in you. You will also be a more competitive applicant for various funding opportunities during your PhD training, as well as in residency, fellowship, and faculty positions. These benefits are not to be overlooked by fellows who have difficulty finding a job, by researchers who have difficulty obtaining grant funding, and considering the increased challenges faced by medical students who do not match to residency or fellowships.

Importantly, in the majority of MD-PhD programs, you will be paid during most or all of your studies. This differs from medical students, who are only paid once they graduate and begin their residency program. While you are leaving some future income on the table (4 years less of working are not necessarily made up for by your MD-PhD stipend), you have the income earlier, allowing you to make it grow with smart investing and a lack of accumulating debt with interest payments.

WHAT SACRIFICES DO YOU MAKE BY JOINING AN MD-PhD PROGRAM?

Enrolling in an MD-PhD program means your training will take a very long time compared to your single-degree MD or PhD colleagues. As stated above, the duration of training, including the MD-PhD program, residency program, and fellowship training, will take 10–15 years. For those who want to quickly graduate and begin earning a doctor's salary, this program is not for them.

For most MD-PhD trainees, there will be some degree of sacrifice in terms of long-term planning of their personal and family lives. For example, most trainees will be moving between multiple institutions throughout the various stages of their training, making family life challenging, while still certainly possible. Many MD-PhD students, including many female trainees, have families at all stages of their MD-PhD program, in residency or afterward.

There is also a degree of risk undertaken in doing an MD-PhD program. Some students will realize that research is not for them, or that they want to continue research in their career, but not in the field they did their PhD in. These risks are important to keep in mind but should not necessarily scare an applicant away from an MD-PhD.

QUICK TIPS FOR STUDENTS WHO RECENTLY ACCEPTED AN MD-PhD PROGRAM OFFER

If you just accepted an offer to an MD-PhD program, congratulations! The first and most important recommendation is to take a bit of time off before starting the first year, to gain some important perspective; it will be a long time until you have this luxury again. The program is seven or more years long, but it flies by quickly.

If you're finishing your current degree program and have an extended summer vacation of several months before starting medical school, it would be wise to get started in a laboratory at your new institution for a few weeks or months in the summer beforehand. This will allow you to begin working on a project and become familiar with the lab environment by getting to know the people in the lab and where reagents are kept. Becoming familiar with the environment will be particularly important if you plan to do research part time during the first year of medical school. Since you will often be coming in on nights and weekends, when it's quiet, you will benefit from having some time to acclimatize yourself to the research environment beforehand, with colleagues to help you.

CONCLUSION

Undertaking joint MD-PhD training can lead to a phenomenal career path that is rewarding and exciting yet challenging. Using the information in this chapter, a reader should be able to come away with a good understanding of what an MD-PhD program entails and for whom such a program is designed. We hope that this information will help in making a decision as to whether you should apply to an MD-PhD program.

2

Choosing the Right MD-PhD Program for You

Mack A. Michell-Robinson

Mack Michell-Robinson *is a third-year MD-PhD student at McGill University. His PhD research is in the field of neurology, focusing on developing experimental models of a rare disease of the central nervous system, along with gene therapies to treat it. Prior to medical school, Mack completed both bachelor's and master of science degrees, and worked as an associate scientist at a Fortune 500 biotechnology company.*

INTRODUCTION

You know you're interested in pursuing an MD-PhD degree, but you're not sure where to start. With over 50 distinct MD-PhD programs in North America, choosing the right program to apply to is a complex decision. Building and submitting a personalized, high-quality application is of paramount importance. There are too many programs to apply to all of them at once!

> **WHAT YOU NEED TO KNOW**
>
> - You must balance academic excellence and life beyond the lab when considering an institution for your MD-PhD studies.
> - There are multiple public resources at your disposal that can help determine the research excellence at an institution. Use publication records and grant funding records to determine how successful a research group and/or department is.
> - Apply to institutions offering the type of training you're interested in, corresponding to the career you want to have.
> - Program funding in the United States is either MSTP or non-MSTP. Both are generous funding packages, but they may have geographical restrictions for applicants and/or different training requirements. Non-MSTP programs may not offer the same funding across all institutions, while MSTP funding packages are generally similar. Don't forget to look at taxation when determining the amount of funds you will have available for living expenses.
> - Internal program funding in Canada varies by institution; meanwhile, external funding opportunities such as federal and provincial scholarships may have additional geographical restrictions.

The first step on the path to an MD-PhD degree is choosing a program in order to build the appropriate application. This chapter and the next aim to help you get started by breaking down the information you need to choose a program and then help you build a winning application by explaining what MD-PhD programs are looking for in candidates.

This chapter will cover important considerations for choosing an MD-PhD program that go beyond choosing a typical medical school program. These include how to evaluate research excellence at an institution or lab of interest, and an introduction to the structuring and financing opportunities available in MD-PhD programs in North America.

ASSESSING RESEARCH EXCELLENCE

We take it for granted that excellence is the primary motivator for an MD-PhD aspirant, so naturally it is appropriate to pick a program that is excellent, too. Unfortunately, academic excellence can be a difficult thing to ascertain before entering a program. All programs have an incentive to portray themselves as excellent to candidates, just as all candidates have an incentive to portray excellence to the programs they apply to. Fortunately, there are a few things applicants can do to learn more about a program and the kind of training they might expect to receive there.

So how do you evaluate the depth and breadth of an institution's research? You'll need to start by looking into the researchers who work there. Running a successful academic lab involves two activities that are subject to public record keeping. These two activities are publishing manuscripts and applying for grant funding. You can use the records of these two activities to do a cursory evaluation of an institution or lab of interest. However, reaching out and networking with the individuals working in the context of a research program can also give you valuable insight about the quality of a research program and the work environment.

Assessing research output using public records

Before trying anything else, I would suggest looking into the recent publications coming from any departments at an institution you find interesting. Look at departmental websites in order to find out which researchers work there, and check their publication record using a publicly available indexing website (e.g., PubMed). I would also recommend looking up a few researchers you find particularly interesting (i.e., potential supervisors) and looking at their h-index using Google Scholar (publicly available) or Web of Science (Clarivate Analytics) if you have access. By looking at the analytics of publication records (e.g., impact factor of journals, number of publications per year, average citations), you will gain insight into the productivity of a research group's membership and the general quality of the research. While analytic approaches to assessing research quality can be flawed, this is certainly the most convenient way to get a big-picture view of research quality and productivity.

Another important consideration is whether a group is well funded. Because grant applications are competitive, successfully obtaining grants is an indicator of the research success that you have access to. Most successful researchers pursue grants from the National Institutes of Health (NIH) in the United States, while Canadian researchers pursue grant funding via the Tri-Council Agencies (CIHR, NSERC, SSHRC). While some departments will periodically publish grant funding numbers, results from the public competitive grant agencies listed above are usually available online. Keep in mind, some research is conducted using private funds, so you will not get the full funding picture from looking at public records. However, a lot of information can be taken away from browsing these records and looking at specific researchers' public grant application success.

Networking

Networking is an important part of picking a research lab once you've started your MD-PhD. If you have the ability to network with people in the departments or labs you're interested in even before applying to an institute, you should. Certainly, you will get the most direct impression of the research excellence at an institute by visiting it and speaking with the people who work there. Interviewing with supervisors to discuss potential research projects and meeting with lab members in those labs and nearby labs is recommended. If you have the opportunity to ask about the career trajectories of past trainees, you will get a picture of what the research training is worth in the broader research community. Furthermore, networking has a number of advantages that go beyond merely assessing the work environment.

Perhaps most importantly, if your networking goes well, you might leave a lasting positive impression on future colleagues or supervisors. You will definitely gain an impression about your potential fit within a department or lab. One of the most commonly asked questions during the MD-PhD admissions interviews is if you have potential supervisors in mind. Being able to respond that you've met several already to discuss research projects will play in your favor with an admissions committee. Networking is invaluable in this respect; having familiarity with potential supervisors and their labs will make it very easy to discuss potential projects in an interview context, and it also gives you the confidence of someone who has the inside scoop.

ASSESSING MEDICAL TRAINING EXCELLENCE

Assessing medical training excellence is difficult because the degree to which doctors succeed in their careers is subjective and hard to track. In order to assess this aspect of a program, it would be a good idea to look at a few sources of medical school rankings (e.g., *Times Higher Education*, *Top Universities*, *Maclean's*). Another method would be to look at the physician-scientists who work at some flagship institutions and see where they trained. If you have physician mentors, it may be a good idea to look into their training background as well. Finally, talking to medical students, residents, or physicians you know may give you additional insight into what they believe is a good place to receive medical training. All of these taken together can help you form a picture of whether or not an institution gives excellent training to medical students.

PROGRAM FORMAT

At North American institutions, formal MD-PhD training generally occurs in one of three configurations over a 7 to 8-year period. Most MD-PhD training programs offer a split curriculum: The PhD portion of the degree is carried out between the pre-clerkship and clerkship years of medical school. Others offer a curriculum format where the PhD and MD are contiguous and are completed one after another. Research residencies and informal completion of both MD and PhD studies fall outside the scope of formal MD-PhD program training but are options as well. Each of these program formats has advantages, which are to be considered when evaluating a training opportunity, and these may be more applicable to some applicants than others. Most if not all institutions employ a variant of one of these general curricular training templates.

Split programs

The most common variant for formal MD-PhD programs is also sometimes called the 2-3-2 or 2-4-2 track or configuration. In a split configuration, the MD program is divided into two parts, most commonly consisting of pre-clerkship (approximately the first 2 years of study) and clerkship years (years 3 and 4). PhD training is completed in between these two parts, after completion of the pre-clerkship training, but before clerkship training. In many programs, especially those in the United States, MD-PhD training opportunities (awards, seminars, and conferences) are available for the full duration of study from the time of matriculation (i.e., year 1). An advantage of this format is that students may have increased access to opportunities that would help evaluate which field of clinical medicine interests them in order to better choose an associated PhD topic. In this regard, the format is appropriate for a wide array of students, including those that have not picked a specific research topic at the time of matriculation. However, as discussed below, many students who successfully matriculate have prior research experience as part of their application package, and that is also a consideration if you value expediency.

Contiguous programs

In the contiguous configuration, students finish graduate studies and subsequently continue to complete a medical school curriculum. In many programs, MD-PhD training opportunities (awards, seminars, conferences) are available for the full duration of study from the time of matriculation in the MD-PhD program. The major advantage of this program structure is that students who have already started graduate studies may be able to translate their ongoing project into MD-PhD studies while taking advantage of augmented funding and training opportunities through the MD-PhD program. Therefore, contiguous programs may be attractive to graduate students whose graduate research is already underway, but who may require additional years to complete it before beginning medical school studies.

Research residencies

Research residencies are a novel format of clinical residency that emphasize research training as a major component of the program requirements. These programs are growing in popularity; however, bear in mind that they may or may not award a doctoral degree at program completion, and they vary in structure on an institutional basis. Most research residencies in the United States follow the standard, field-specific residency training format for the first 1 to 2 years, followed by a modified schedule that allocates anywhere from 50% to 90% of time to research. The duration of the total time in residency varies. In Canada, research residencies are offered at many institutions through the Clinician Investigator Program, which provides a funding package to cover additional research training.

Research residency programs may be appropriate for excellent medical students with limited research experience who are interested in pursuing or participating in a research program as part of their career, or those with specific research interests in their desired field of medicine. Additionally, a research residency could be appropriate for an MD-PhD program graduate interested in obtaining time to pursue postdoctoral research during residency training. In sum, research residencies are a good choice for medical residents who have completed their MD program and want to increase involvement in research activities prior to completion of residency.

Non-MD-PhD program training

Students may complete medical and graduate training entirely separately, although this is not recommended, as it forgoes the advantages of an integrated program structure, such as reduced total time of study and increased funding and training opportunities. It can, however, be advantageous to students nearly finished with a current doctorate training program.

WHEN DO I WRITE THE USMLE IN A SPLIT MD-PhD PROGRAM?

In my case, I have elected to write the Step One exam at the end of my PhD studies to avoid an issue with the United States Medical Licensing Examination (USMLE) window. Details of the USMLE are covered in Chapter 21, so it will not be discussed in further detail here. It is important to remember to take deadlines and expiration dates for all standardized exams into account when planning your educational trajectory. However, USMLE scheduling is not likely to be a major consideration when choosing an accredited MD-PhD program.

PROGRAM FUNDING AND COSTS

As with other graduate studies in science, technology, engineering, and medicine, funds are generally supplied to students to defray the cost of tuition and/or living expenses during MD-PhD studies. Funding for students pursuing MD-PhD studies varies both between institutions and between the US and Canada, as do the costs associated with attending a given institution. Most institutions post up-to-date figures concerning funding for students on their website, taking into consideration the costs of enrollment and approximate costs of living. Here we will cover the fundamentals of the funding structures for MD-PhD programs, but one should always evaluate the specific funding structures and opportunities in a given program of study. When evaluating a program, special attention should be paid to program funding, as differences in both funds and costs can translate into significant sums saved or spent over the 7 to 8-year training period.

Program funding and costs—USA

In the United States, the NIH provides applicable MD-PhD programs called Medical Scientist Training Programs (MSTP) with significant funds to cover students' tuition/fees and stipends for the full duration of study. The Ruth L. Kirschstein National Research Service Award Institutional Research Training Grant confers on forty-eight institutions the ability to administer MSTP awards to MD-PhD matriculants. This means that applicable MD-PhD program costs in the United States are completely or almost completely covered by the NIH, in addition to a guaranteed stipend for living expenses. These awards are not loans, and students incur no direct debt obligation as a result of accepting them. Additionally, further funding is available through competitive application to NRSA predoctoral training funding opportunities, which can be pursued with a supervisor during study. Non-MSTP MD-PhD programs usually offer similar financial support through institutional funds, with some variation between institutions. Finally, MSTP training opportunities are restricted to citizens or nationals of the United States or those previously admitted for permanent residency. Non-MSTP funding opportunities might be available to matriculants from other countries, which is of special relevance to dual citizens and other foreign nationals.

Program funding and costs—Canada

In Canada, MD-PhD funding has a more complex landscape. Funds for training generally come from institutional scholarships and provincial or federal funding agencies. Provincial or federal awards are now generally apportioned for research training only (i.e., MSc, PhD, or postdoctoral study), so they can rarely be used to fund the first 2 years of medicine in split programs. Programs that provide guaranteed support for the complete duration of MD-PhD study, such as the one at McGill University, often do so out of dedicated institutional funds. Government training awards superimpose an even greater degree of complexity, discussed below. Although these awards are available, they must be obtained through competition. Therefore, if considering MD-PhD training in Canada, it is especially important to take into account internal funding and support resources available at a given institution, because external funding is never completely guaranteed.

Significant external provincial or federal awards are usually available to students with Canadian citizenship through competitive application processes; MD-PhD students, along with other graduate students, are eligible to apply for such funding (Canadian Institutes of Health Research [CIHR], etc.) for the PhD portion of training. Although highly competitive, many of these awards are quite lucrative. Two examples include the Vanier Scholarship and the doctoral awards offered by the Tri-Council Agencies. Numerous provincial awards exist that have similar funding schema for doctoral research. For example, in Quebec the Fonds de Recherche de Santé Québec (FRSQ) offers a doctoral training award competition specifically to MD-PhD students.

In Canada, as a general rule, more than one major scholarship cannot be held at the same time so that funds can be accessed by more students (i.e., they are not "stackable"). Furthermore, institutional (internal) funding in Canada usually guarantees only a minimum stipend; so if external funding is obtained in addition to an institutional stipend, it may not augment the total amount of a student's funding unless the amounts awarded externally exceed the minimum stipend amount. External funding, such as federal or provincial training awards, are likely to be the most lucrative option for MD-PhD candidates during the research years of their degree; and funds can continue to be used as long as research continues (up to the limit of the duration of the award). Overall, these awards are accessible for most MD-PhD candidates at top institutions and should be evaluated as a key part of any MD-PhD funding considerations.

FUNDING YOUR MD-PhD TRAINING

Funding for MD-PhD training is a critical consideration when evaluating programs of study. In general, MD-PhD training in the United States is comprehensively funded and comes with little to no associated tuition cost. However, living expenses in many areas can be significant, and prospective students ought to consider mechanisms for reducing these expenses in addition to funds awarded at a given institute when evaluating programs of interest. Furthermore, the issue of taxation on awards offered by institutions in the United States will vary at the state and federal level over time and may significantly impact living expenses, especially if tuition rebates are counted as income. It is especially important to speak with the financial aid office and an accountant in order to come to conclusions about what a funding package really offers.

In Canadian training programs, funding schemes vary significantly by institution and seldom cover tuition costs. However, tuition itself as well as living costs can be a fraction of those in the United States and may be less of a factor when evaluating total debt incurred through study. Most or all of these costs may be covered through institutional, provincial, or federal awards obtained through competitive application processes.

In either country, it is also worth noting that financial institutions generally look favorably on lending lines of credit to medical students, and MD-PhD students are equally considered under this umbrella in most cases. Therefore, individuals applying to MD-PhD programs in either country must think about funding, tuition, and living expenses as key features in evaluating the financial feasibility of training over a 7 to 8-year period.

DOES A PROGRAM FIT ME?

Fit is a difficult concept to describe, because it is completely subjective—it is the integration of everything we talk about in these chapters and how it adds to, or subtracts from, your life during the program. In a way, fit is difficult to evaluate because it is gestalt—living life as an MD-PhD student and fitting into your program is more than just the sum of the individual parts you think about when evaluating a program. To assess fit, it can help to prioritize based on things that make you happy, that make you feel content in your work, and that make you confident in your approach to pursuing the career of your dreams.

Reflecting on what is important to you will also identify how well your personal values and motives align with an institution you are applying to. Life experiences that may have brought you difficulty or hardship are equally important in evaluating fit, because avoiding something you dislike is an important decision, too. If there are things you know you need, make sure they are provided for. For example, one aspect of my master's training environment that I enjoyed was that it was next door to the fitness center at my school. I valued having the ability to stay healthy without sacrificing working hours. The fitness I was able to maintain helped further my productivity without any strain on the other aspects of my life. Sometimes values are difficult to know consciously, and gut feelings are okay where fit is concerned.

As an exercise, you may want to make a spreadsheet outlining features of your candidate schools that align with your own personal values and goals. On this spreadsheet, you can fill in specific items that promote your own personal happiness and productivity, assigning weight to how important each of these features is. Doing this will help you more concretely understand what might be important features that your target schools should have. You can then compare these items to those emphasized by different institutions. The absence of these soft aspects of a potential program could be a deal breaker, depending on how much weight you place on each aspect. Will your research be valued where you work? Are students treated well by supervisors in the program? Are there others like you who are happy with their decision to attend the program? Would you feel good about your future job prospects as a result of entering a program? You will notice that these are all examples of subjective and personal responses you might have to a particular environment you may be interested in.

As previously discussed, it is always a good idea to reach out to people in the programs you're applying to, attend open houses or events, and read promotional materials. Each of these things will give you a different feeling for how you might fit into a given program, institution, or lab. Never overlook fit when evaluating an opportunity.

LIFE BEYOND THE LAB

This aspect of the program you intend to pick is often pushed to the bottom of the list when considering programs of interest, but I urge you not to do that. Not only is your life beyond the lab a critical aspect of how you fit into a program, but it may turn out to be these aspects of life during the program that drive or sink your productivity. Assume for a second that you do get a position in your favorite school, but life there just isn't what you expected. You go through difficult training circumstances each day, faced with the trials and tribulations of mastering not one new vocation, but two. In your moments of free time, wouldn't you prefer to enjoy yourself and be energized by it?

Considerations for life beyond the lab include your social network; nearby family and friends made prior to medical school can be an incredible source of support and a necessary oasis in the midst of MD-PhD training. It's also important to evaluate the locale where the school is situated. Neighborhood safety, affordability, and accessibility are all valid concerns. You may find you have less free time than anticipated in an MD-PhD program, and it would be a shame to spend it stuck in traffic.

In terms of leisure activities, does the school provide mechanisms for social integration and all-important fun? Maybe you enjoy sports or artistic pursuits—does the school have programs, groups, or meetups that could provide an outside social network while you are doing your favorite hobby? Finally, an important consideration for any student in a difficult professional degree program is mental health. Many schools offer resources that are free of charge to help you deal with stressful, unforeseen circumstances. These resources should be evaluated in addition to the ones mentioned above, because they can be critical in times of need. Whatever is at your disposal to keep you on track, well, and focused is important to investigate before you submit your application.

CONCLUSION

Pursuing an MD-PhD program is a large commitment, and choosing an institution with a program that promotes your success throughout your studies is critical. I have explained how to assess a program's academic merit and highlighted the advantages and disadvantages of different program formats. Beyond that, you should be considering academic excellence, life beyond the lab, opportunities for extracurricular activities, and program fit.

Each of these elements depends greatly on the needs of the applicant, of course. Reflect on which elements are most valuable to you, as this reflection will allow you to choose programs that fit best and promote your success throughout your MD-PhD studies and beyond.

3

Positioning Yourself for a Successful MD-PhD Application

Chirag Vasavda • Jared Hinkle

Chirag Vasavda *entered the MD-PhD program at Johns Hopkins University in 2014. He joined the Biochemistry, Cellular and Molecular Biology graduate program and studied under Dr. Solomon Snyder in the Department of Neuroscience. In graduate school, he discovered that the heme metabolite bilirubin binds and activates the orphan receptor MRGPRX4 in itch sensory neurons, potentially contributing to itch in hepatobiliary disease. He also identified that bilirubin is a physiologic antioxidant with distinct redox activity that negatively regulates superoxide signaling during neurotransmission.*

Jared Hinkle *entered the MD-PhD program at Johns Hopkins University in 2015 and joined the Department of Neuroscience graduate program in 2017. He is conducting his PhD thesis research in the laboratories of Drs. Ted and Valina Dawson and is currently investigating how glial cells respond to fibrillar α-synuclein in Parkinson's disease.*

WHAT YOU NEED TO KNOW

- MD-PhD programs want to train future physician-scientists—your application should make it clear that you aspire to be one.
- MD-PhD programs are looking for individuals who have a track record of academic success and who demonstrate intellectual curiosity. They will be looking for a rigorous academic program that is broad but also focused on your specific interests, and they will evaluate your GPA and MCAT scores as part of your application.
- Admissions committees are looking for applications that express empathy, a propensity toward service, and a sense of duty to care for others.
- Research is at the heart of a physician-scientist's career, and your application must demonstrate a serious commitment to it. The strongest applicants have extensive research experiences in which they have made meaningful contributions. You do not have to have publications to demonstrate that.
- Keep track of research opportunities and supervisors to refer to when you need letters of recommendation that reinforce your promise as a physician-scientist and point to specific experiences and contributions as evidence.

INTRODUCTION

Applying to any advanced degree program requires coordinating and juggling a complex set of requirements and deadlines. While some of these requirements are more straightforward and obvious, others may feel nebulous, intimidating, and even exhausting. For students applying to MD-PhD programs, it can feel like the maze of applying to medical school only worsens the complexities of applying to graduate school. Here, we outline what MD-PhD admissions committees look for, so that you can prepare now to build a competitive application in the future. While some programs may value different aspects of the application, we lay out the basic principles of what program committees seek in their future students. Essentially, MD-PhD admissions committees are guided by a clear mission: to train future physician-scientists. Accordingly, they are looking for evidence that you can live up to that charge. We also recommend you read Chapters 6 and 7, on the building of your application and the application process, to get a better idea of how the efforts described here will strengthen your final application once you are actually applying. They offer some advice that will be helpful even this early in your preparation.

MD-PhD PROGRAMS WANT TO TRAIN FUTURE PHYSICIAN-SCIENTISTS

Being a physician-scientist is more than the sum of its parts. MD-PhD programs are not just looking to train physicians who do research or scientists who care for patients. Instead, programs are seeking to train individuals who can bridge the worlds of clinical medicine, research, and teaching. As a result, the nature of applying to MD-PhD programs shares some similarities with applying to MD or PhD programs separately, but also differs in significant ways.

Because MD-PhD programs combine medical and graduate training, they are also long and rigorous. This requires trainees to be truly committed not only to succeed during training, but also to thrive in their careers as independent physician-scientists. Specifically, a successful MD-PhD applicant will demonstrate academic success in undergraduate coursework and standardized testing, a passion for clinical medicine and service, and a commitment to research. Your potential as a future physician-scientist will be evident not only in your academic achievements and experiences, but also reinforced in letters of recommendation and personal statements.

ACADEMIC SUCCESS

Rigor, breadth, and depth

Just as with applying to medical school, most MD-PhD programs will require you to complete certain coursework. These prerequisites will vary from school to school, but in general you will need to take courses in biology, general chemistry, organic chemistry, physics, math, statistics, humanities, social science, and behavioral science. These courses will help you lay a foundation to build upon in medical and graduate school.

Some schools will accept Advanced Placement (AP) or International Baccalaureate (IB) credits in order to satisfy some of the prerequisites, but not all schools do. Because the policies vary so widely across institutions, it is generally safer to incorporate the required courses as part of your undergraduate or postbaccalaureate academic program.

Although the prerequisite coursework is itself challenging, MD-PhD programs also look for students who challenge themselves with additional rigorous and stimulating courses.

Because being a physician-scientist requires a thirst for and a commitment to learning, admissions committees are looking for signs that you pushed yourself to advance your learning. Admissions committees recognize and appreciate students who build a broad base of knowledge, but also when students dive deep into their interests through research or advanced coursework. They will assess how you engaged with your academic environment in college to paint a picture of your interests, curiosity, and academic potential. For example, junior or senior students could consider enrolling in honors or, if available, graduate courses that interest them. Graduate-level coursework not only serves as an experience for students to preview what might lie ahead during graduate school, but is also an opportunity to demonstrate intellectual curiosity and academic readiness to admissions committees. Academic projects outside your curriculum like writing, coding, and teaching can also help admissions committees formulate a picture of your ambitions and motivations.

However, there are certain practical limitations to the detail with which your coursework experience will be scrutinized. For example, the individuals reviewing your application will largely rely upon the reputation of your undergraduate institution and the titles of your courses to infer the type of formal education experience that you have received. It is not likely that they will be intimately familiar with the courses themselves or their specific content. While taking an honors version of organic chemistry may be viewed as a distinction, less explicitly leveled structures (e.g., "easy" calculus 201 versus "hard" calculus 301) will probably not be perceived. As such, it can be helpful to strategize how you fulfill general requirements in a manner that will not unnecessarily distract from your time to pursue extracurriculars or ability to earn acceptable grades.

Grades

Admissions committees will use your grade point average (GPA) to roughly measure your success within your academic program. Many MD-PhD programs publish the range or average GPAs of their entering class on their websites. Often these GPA ranges are not absolute minimums but rather yardsticks designed to give you an idea of the profile of the typical candidate who was accepted to that particular MD-PhD program. While some schools do have explicit minimum GPAs, most programs do not triage applications by GPA. Instead, they holistically review each application.

Having good grades is nonetheless extremely important, and successful MD-PhD applicants tend to have higher GPAs than their MD- and PhD-only counterparts. The Association of American Medical Colleges (AAMC) details metrics for incoming MD and MD-PhD applicants and matriculants that are publicly accessible, which may be helpful when gauging your competitiveness in either sphere. Generally, applicants with GPAs below 3.5 are less likely to receive interview invitations, but admissions committees may recognize the limitations of the GPA in evaluating candidates, including: (1) GPAs are an imprecise measure of academic capability that are often not comparable across majors or institutions; (2) Students who take less challenging courses may have higher GPAs than applicants who took more challenging or higher-level courses; (3) GPAs can crudely and harshly penalize students who dealt with periods of adversity or students whose academic performance improved over time. As such, do not be entirely dissuaded from applying if your GPA is lower than you'd like because you got off to a slow start, especially if you did much better in your later courses or if life circumstances explain a period of poor performance.

Applicants often view GPAs as one of the more ambiguous and frustrating components of their application for several reasons. Firstly, GPAs are not necessarily comparable across students. GPAs also don't fully capture a student's complete academic successes or future potential. Moreover, there are sometimes more applicants with extremely high or near-perfect GPAs to a program than there are spots, rendering the GPA useless in differentiating these applicants. In these instances, a high GPA will not set you apart from other applicants, but a low GPA can hurt your chances of admission. For these reasons and others, admissions committees often look to standardized tests like the Medical College Admission Test (MCAT) for additional insight into an applicant's academic potential.

Standardized tests

Nearly all MD-PhD programs require applicants to take the MCAT, with few to no exceptions. The process of preparing for and taking the exam will be more extensively covered in the next chapter, but the test is important enough to also be addressed here. Another standardized test, the Computer-based Assessment for Sampling Personal Characteristics (CASPer), may also be part of your application process. See Chapter 5 for details on preparing for that assessment.

The MCAT is a standardized, multiple-choice, computer-based exam that tests knowledge in four broad categories: biological and biochemical foundations of living systems; chemical and physical foundations of biological systems; psychological, social, and biological foundations of behavior; and critical analysis and reasoning skills. MD-PhD programs also do not require the Graduate Record Examination (GRE).

Many programs use the MCAT to contextualize and understand an applicant's GPA and academic achievements, since it is a more standardized academic assessment than the GPA. Accordingly, it is important to do well on the MCAT. As with GPAs, many programs publish the range or average MCAT score of their entering class on their websites. While few MD-PhD programs in the United States publicize minimum MCAT scores, programs in Canada commonly require a minimum score in order to apply.

Begin preparing for the MCAT by first working backwards to identify when you will take the exam. Students commonly take the MCAT in the calendar year before they plan to matriculate in medical school, but many take it earlier. It is usually worthwhile to take the MCAT early enough to know your score before you submit your application. Let's imagine a case in which you plan to matriculate in medical school next August. In this case, you'll be submitting your primary application in the prior summer (typically June or July). In order to receive your MCAT score before you submit your primary application, you would want to take your MCAT before April of the year you plan to apply, so that you receive your score in May or June, before you apply. If you think you may need to take the exam more than once, you'll want to consider taking the MCAT well before. You can take the MCAT multiple times, and many schools explicitly state that they will consider your highest overall score.

Next, identify the material you will be tested on. The content and format of the MCAT constantly evolves, so it's useful to take some time to review the most current information provided by the AAMC regarding the MCAT. Regardless of format, the MCAT will likely test material that is typically covered in introductory-level biology, general and organic chemistry, biochemistry, physics, psychology, human physiology, and sociology courses. While having a broad base of biomedical knowledge is an advantage, it is important to recognize that the MCAT tests material in applied contexts using questions based on short passages. For a minority of questions, you will simply need to have the requisite background knowledge, but the majority of its questions can technically be answered by correctly interpreting the content of the passages. Because of this, the MCAT is in part a test of mental stamina and of processing new information in a quick and effective manner. In order to earn a competitive score, you need both an exceptional depth of content familiarity and extensive practice with test-taking. As such, most students find that taking practice exams at a simulated exam pace is the most effective way to push their score into the upper percentiles.

Lastly, give yourself enough time to prepare for the exam. It is important to take the exam only when you are prepared and ready. Be sure you are comfortable with the content and format of the exam. There are several free and low-cost resources available to help you review content and test yourself. The AAMC offers official MCAT preparation tools and resources on their website to help you familiarize yourself with the format of the exam. Similarly, organizations like Khan Academy have developed free online video lectures and tutorials.

Pace yourself—studying for the MCAT is a marathon, not a sprint.

PASSION FOR CLINICAL MEDICINE AND SERVICE

In addition to academic success, a strong MD-PhD applicant has extensive experience volunteering and shadowing within the health care system. Just like their MD-only classmates, MD-PhD students are also training to be physicians who care for patients. It is essential that your application conveys an understanding of the intersection between science and medicine and a desire to pursue a career as a practicing physician. This is especially important at institutions where students must first be accepted into the medical school before they are considered for admission to the combined MD-PhD program.

Medical schools and MD-PhD admissions committees will evaluate your clinical experience by the length and depth of your commitment, the diversity of your experiences, and the lessons you've learned from the experiences. Students can gain clinical experience through various volunteer services or shadowing. Volunteering at clinics and hospitals will expose you to diverse health care settings with teams of providers and are more valued than isolated volunteer experiences such as "voluntourism." Chapter 6 ("Building Your MD-PhD Application") breaks down the volunteer experiences that make for the strongest application.

In contrast, shadowing a physician may offer you insight into life as a doctor and provide details about specific specializations and fields. Admissions committees are also aware that some applicants are not always able to shadow or volunteer during the academic year. Most programs tend to evaluate students based on the opportunities they had and what they did with them, and admissions committees deeply appreciate the students who sought out opportunities to volunteer or shadow when they could.

Social awareness

Significant evidence suggests that a complex interplay of social, economic, and political determinants shapes patients' overall health alongside access to medical care. As a result, physicians must be increasingly familiar and fluent in seeing a patient's health beyond just a biomedical problem and instead as the sum of biological and social factors. Deep inequities exist among patients, with socioeconomic, physical, and behavioral variables contributing to dramatic differences between patients' well-being. For example, Americans with low socio-economic status develop illnesses in their thirties and forties that patients of higher status only present with several decades later. There are also various additional inequities that exist, making the causes of these disparities more complex than simply socioeconomic status.

Being fluent in the language of social determinants of health requires social awareness and an understanding of how education, income, nutrition, racism (institutional or otherwise), implicit bias, and housing policy influence health. Admissions committees are looking for applications that express empathy, a propensity toward service, and a sense of duty to care for others. They are looking to train individuals who value all people regardless of race, sexual orientation, ethnicity, socioeconomic status, religion, or other differences. Admissions committees look at your volunteering, political involvement, charity work, or activism as windows into your compassion and humanity.

COMMITMENT TO RESEARCH

Research is at the heart of a physician-scientist's career, but many medical schools are beginning to focus earlier on clinical care and requiring larger numbers of classes. Accordingly, it will be increasingly difficult for those who pursue only an MD to conduct independent basic or translational research while in medical school. The gap between scientists and physicians is expected to grow within the current structure of academic medicine. Your application must demonstrate a serious commitment to the complementary education of both MD and PhD degrees and a desire to bridge this expanding gap. A research statement, personal narrative, or both may be required and are your opportunity to show that you are the perfect candidate. Chapters 6 and 7, on the building and submission of your application, address this topic further.

The most compelling applicants have extensive research experiences in which they have made meaningful contributions to the lab or project. If you plan to study basic or applied experimental science in graduate school, then prior experience in an experimental laboratory is essential. Similarly, if you are considering pursuing a PhD outside the laboratory sciences, it will be just as important to demonstrate familiarity and experience with the discipline. In general, successful MD-PhD applicants spend 10–20 hours per week in lab during the academic year and transition to full time during the summers.

Early in your bachelor's degree, you can declare an honors-program major with a year or more research component that provides access to a lab. While it is not necessary that you begin working in a lab your first semester freshman year of college, the earlier and longer you are involved in research, the better. Many programs will not be convinced of your commitment to research if you have fewer than two semesters of experience in the lab before you apply. However, demonstrating commitment to research does not require post-graduate research experience, and students with substantial research experience in undergraduate school are often admitted directly without more years of research required. It is valuable to experience different research environments, but not required; having many distinct short experiences at the expense of deeper involvement is unwise. There is no right answer to the question "How much lab experience is ideal?" However, it takes time to learn the techniques and background science that allow a subsequent focus on learning to think like a scientist.

While summer laboratory experiences can be helpful in exposing you to different areas of research, summers are generally too short to make substantive contributions to the lab. As a result, programs value research experiences that are continuous with the same lab over multiple semesters. By committing to a single or a few labs during your undergraduate or post-baccalaureate academic program, you'll not only mature in your knowledge of the research, but you will be more capable of making meaningful contributions to the work. That is not to say that summer research experiences cannot be valuable. If there are limited opportunities to pursue research at your school or in your area, don't hesitate to apply to summer programs elsewhere. A summer research experience at another institution can also expose you to an area of research not available locally or allow you to explore a new field of research without committing to a full semester or more. Spending enough time in the lab is not just important for your application, but also for yourself to help you decide whether this really is for you.

Your research experience itself and your contributions are the most important products from your time in the lab. While publications might be more tangible than experiences, MD-PhD admissions committees are hyper-aware that publications are often require the right circumstances and luck, as well as hard work and acumen. First-, second-, and middle-author publications are not required for admission to MD-PhD programs, and the vast majority of students are admitted without any publications. Admissions committees are not looking for a publication record, but instead a demonstrated commitment to the pursuit of science, a familiarity with the process of discovery, and the unique intellectual and emotional challenges that a career in science entails.

LETTERS OF RECOMMENDATION

Most MD-PhD admissions committees request letters from your professors and mentors that speak to your credentials and abilities. Because applicants spend years developing and completing the credentials needed to apply to MD-PhD programs, letters of recommendation may seem like a small and insignificant element of the application. Their importance might also be overlooked because most applicants do not seek letters until the final stages of the application process.

That said, their significance cannot be overstated. Admissions committees rely on letters of recommendation to help them paint a better overall picture of your accomplishments, potential, and character. Chapter 7 outlines the necessary elements of a strong recommendation letter, but it is worth considering potential references even now. Good letters of recommendation will support and corroborate your application, whereas lukewarm or negative letters can be ruinous. Great letters can inspire admissions committees to see the person you are and your potential as a physician-scientist. You're looking for someone to give a glowing account of your research contributions, but you may also want a reference to strengthen your application in a specific way. Keep track of your research opportunities, supervisors, and your experience with them, so you can easily refer to those records when considering who to contact for a proper letter of recommendation.

The requirements for the numbers and types of letters vary widely, so it is worthwhile to take the time to identify any particularities among the schools to which you are applying. Typically, MD admissions committees will want to hear from two faculty members in science departments who have taught you and one non-science faculty member. These letters should be written by faculty members and not by graduate students, postdoctoral fellows, or teaching assistants. However, a letter from a senior faculty member who does not know you is not helpful. To ensure that you are presented in the best possible light, solicit letters from professors and advisors who will enthusiastically advocate for you. Ideally, your letters should provide concrete examples, vivid vignettes, and sincere emotion. These letters are also typically confidential, or at least submitted independently by the writer, so you will most likely not have an opportunity to suggest changes or additions to the letter. For this reason, it is important to choose faculty who know you well and to explicitly ask the writers whether they think they can independently write you a supportive letter. In addition to providing peace of mind, this can helpfully prompt a discussion of your aspirations and accomplishments.

MD-PhD programs specifically require a letter from at least one of your research mentors and expect a letter from anyone with whom you worked for more than a few months. This letter is possibly one of the most important dimensions of your application. As for selecting who writes your letters, admissions committees prefer to hear from the principal investigator, or the senior-most individual who advised you. They should provide specific examples of your contributions to the lab and highlight your scientific growth. Most importantly, this letter should inspire confidence in your scientific acumen, your enthusiasm for research, and your interest in medicine. In situations where the principal investigator cannot write a meaningful letter alone, it might be helpful if they were to write a letter together with whoever mentored you directly. While the credentials of the person who writes this letter do matter, it matters far more what the letter says about you.

CONCLUSION

Applying to MD-PhD programs may feel daunting, but the opportunities that lie ahead of it make it worthwhile. Programs are looking for students who demonstrate that they are ready for and sincerely seek those opportunities. In principle, admissions committees admit students who demonstrate three characteristics: academic excellence, a passion for clinical medicine, and a commitment to research. A history of academic success is critical for both medical and graduate training, since both careers require extensive class time, testing, and a lifelong commitment to learning. MD-PhD programs are also training students who want to become both physicians and scientists. Accordingly, your application should convey an understanding of the intersection between science and medicine through significant clinical and research experiences.

Despite the high standards, successfully applying to MD-PhD programs is well within reach. There are many MD-PhD programs across the United States and Canada, many of which admit 10–25-plus students per year. Of the tens of thousands of students who apply to MD programs each year, less than 5% are applying to MD-PhD programs. Over a third of those MD-PhD applicants receive an offer for admission. By positioning yourself early for a successful MD-PhD application, you will be well on your way to becoming a physician-scientist.

4

Standardized Testing—The MCAT

Sarah Maritan • Joan Miguel Romero • Mark Sorin

Sarah Maritan *is a first-year student in McGill University's MD-PhD program. She received her bachelor of science degree in life sciences and her master of science degree in pathology and molecular medicine from Queen's University in Kingston, Ontario. Her research focuses on the cellular signaling mechanisms regulating cancer progression, particularly the pathways underlying tumor cell movement and metastatic growth.*

Joan Miguel Romero *is a first-year MD-PhD student at McGill University. He completed his honors bachelor of science degree in pathobiology and immunology and his master of science degree in laboratory medicine and pathobiology at the University of Toronto. His research is aimed at understanding the anti-tumor immune mechanisms involved in pancreatic cancer.*

Mark Sorin *is a first-year MD-PhD student at McGill University. He graduated with a bachelor of science in pharmacology from McGill University, where he studied the immune pathways underlying the pathogenesis of asthma. He is currently conducting research in the fields of lung cancer and immunotherapies.*

INTRODUCTION

A rite of passage for generations of physicians past, the MCAT represents the first standardized exam of your future medical career. The majority of medical schools in Canada and the United States use this exam as a screening threshold for medical school applications. As such, it is important that you are familiar with the exam, study well, and get a competitive score. In this chapter, we will outline what this exam entails and provide studying resource

WHAT YOU NEED TO KNOW

- The Medical College Admission Test (MCAT) is an exam administered by the Association of American Medical Colleges (AAMC).
- It is a computerized exam used in the medical admissions process, testing your basic knowledge of biology, chemistry, physics, psychology, and analysis and reasoning skills.
- When you should take the MCAT depends on your academic stage, your preparedness, and other considerations, including time you can dedicate for studying.
- Studying for this exam includes dedicated courses, study guides, and online resources, including practice exams.
- Preparing for the MCAT will give you a glimpse of the dedication and perseverance required to study for the first of many standardized medical exams.

suggestions that we used when we studied for the exam. We then conclude the chapter with what to expect the day of the exam and afterward.

MEDICAL COLLEGE ADMISSION TEST (MCAT)

What is the MCAT?

The Medical College Admission Test (MCAT) is a standardized, multiple-choice exam administered by the Association of American Medical Colleges (AAMC) and is a required component of applications to many medical schools in the United States and Canada. The test is designed to assess your knowledge and critical-thinking skills in a variety of areas. It is divided into four sections: (1) Chemical and Physical Foundations of Biological Systems, (2) Critical Analysis and Reasoning Skills, (3) Biological and Biochemical Foundations of Living Systems, and (4) Psychological, Social, and Biological Foundations of Behavior. Many schools publicize what they consider to be a minimum, average, or competitive MCAT score on their websites, and it is certainly worthwhile doing some research into the schools to which you are applying. In this chapter, we will discuss our personal experiences with the MCAT, including different timelines we followed, various ways to prepare, and suggestions for the exam day itself.

When should you take the MCAT?

Given that you've decided you will be taking the MCAT, the second most important consideration is when. The majority of candidates apply to medical school during their undergraduate degree, and a growing percentage of students now apply after graduation, during postgraduate work or graduate school. First, we will discuss when it is best to take the MCAT during your undergraduate degree, followed by a discussion of taking the exam during graduate school. We will also discuss some logistical considerations regarding when to schedule your exam in the year.

Taking the MCAT during an undergraduate degree

During a typical 4-year premedical undergraduate program, the first 2 years build a strong foundation for biology, physiology, anatomy, chemistry, and physics, with some biochemistry and elective courses on the humanities. For this reason, many students opt to take the MCAT shortly after (or even during) their second year, since they have recently completed these prerequisite courses, and the information is relatively fresh. Another advantage of taking the exam at this time is that, assuming you are applying to enter medical school after fourth year, it gives you the opportunity to retake the exam prior to another cycle of applications, if you wish to improve your score. Other students may opt to take the exam the year of applying to medical school, which is also a reasonable choice. However, it is important to consider that if you take the exam during this time, you must also manage medical school applications concurrently, and must therefore manage your time well.

Taking the MCAT during a graduate degree

Taking the MCAT during graduate school is certainly possible without taking substantial time away from laboratory duties. While every graduate program is different in terms of deadlines and timelines, we believe that the key component to juggling lab work and MCAT preparation is twofold: first, to treat studying like your evening and weekend job, and second, to have a graduate supervisor who is aware and supportive of your plans to take the exam.

The part-time study approach, where your evenings and weekends become designated MCAT study time, is one often adopted by graduate students. It is important to schedule your MCAT at a point in your graduate program that enables you to have your evenings and weekends relatively free for studying. For most, this ideal time is likely in the earlier stages of a degree, before experiments ramp up and thesis deadlines loom. However, others may find that it may be better suited toward the end of a degree, where a majority of work is data analysis that can be done remotely. This is a personal choice and is certainly something to discuss with your supervisor.

It is important to note that this part-time study approach will require a lengthier preparation time than your peers who have the flexibility to study full time, as it involves putting in fewer study hours each day, but over a longer time frame. Furthermore, this approach requires a lot of discipline, as your usual relaxation time will now be filled with more work. In the week or two leading up to the exam, it may be worthwhile to take some time off from lab duties (hence the importance of having a supportive supervisor!), in order to catch up on some material and to take some full-length practice tests, which require a full day's commitment.

Logistical considerations

As the MCAT is administered by the AAMC, the exam scheduling is done through the AAMC website. Annually, there are usually two exam dates in January and approximately four in the spring, with the majority being in the summer months, from June to early September. The exam schedule is usually released in February of each year, and it is worthwhile booking your examination date as early as possible, as prices will increase if you book close to your that date. In addition to elevated prices, spots are limited and will fill up. Booking your exam at the last minute may leave you with limited locations available, which may result in additional travel costs (and stress!). Early booking helps avoid such challenges.

The length of time required to study for the MCAT will depend both on your educational background and what stage of career you are in when applying. The majority of testing dates are in the summer, and it is common that students choose to study during the early summer months and take the exam toward the end of summer. However, this timeline is not suited for everyone, and there are many factors to consider. Do you have an educational background in any of the exam content? Can you block off a few months, or are you going to be working while studying? If so, is it full-time or part-time work? Do you want to have any time off after taking the exam? It is important to pick a schedule that works for your particular situation, being sure not to fall behind on any other work or research-related duties, and of course being sure to take time for life outside of studying to prevent burnout. It is often recommended to block off a week or two immediately prior to the exam to dedicate to full-time reviewing.

When you book the test, there are two important dates to make note of: the date of the actual exam and the date when the results will be released. You must pay attention to both of these dates; make sure that the testing date is suitable for you but also that the accompanying score release date fits the deadlines of the schools to which you are applying. Do you want to know your score before applying, or are you willing to submit the scores blindly to the schools? Do you want to leave yourself time to retake the exam after finding out your score? These are factors to consider when booking your test. Be particularly careful to look into deadlines for combined programs, such as MD-PhD programs. These may have unique application deadlines compared to a school's MD-only program.

Ultimately, when you take the MCAT depends on your learning style, your current stage in your academic training, and most importantly, how prepared you feel. Regardless of when you decide to take it, it is an exciting point in your training, as it represents the first standardized test from a long list of many that you must complete during your path to become a licensed physician.

PREPARING FOR THE MCAT

Taking courses

An important consideration when preparing for the MCAT is whether or not to take preparatory courses. These courses often include lecture-style classes with assignments, study textbooks, and practice questions. The decision of whether or not to take a course depends on your learning style. For those who can actively learn from a textbook and study best in an independent fashion, a course might not be necessary. A course might be a good idea for those who prefer having assignments and a tutor explain concepts to them during scheduled class time.

In terms of picking a course, one needs to consider several factors such as cost, which preparatory material is included, and whether class time fits with one's schedule. Reviews of the course by fellow classmates can also be beneficial when deciding whether a course is right for you. Cost can be a significant barrier to signing up for a course, as some can run upward of a few thousand dollars. Certain university student-run clubs auction MCAT preparatory courses at a reduced price compared to the actual value of said course, a viable solution to reduce costs.

One of the advantages of taking a course is that it provides a structure from which one can study more easily. In addition, many tips are shared with students who take the course. For someone with a part-time job or other obligations, a course can help to stay on track. Overall, your method of learning should guide your decisions on whether an MCAT preparatory course is right for you.

Buying books (or not!)

Whether you decide to take a course or not, you also have the option of using additional resources to study for the exam. Several companies offer their own iterations of preparation for the exam, each with features that are unique to that company/book. Further, depending on how you feel about particular subjects, you also have the option of buying single-subject books or entire sets.

For example, if you have a typical premedical background, you may feel fairly strong on biology or biochemistry, and rather than buying a complete set covering all subjects tested on the MCAT, you may buy select books on subjects you are less familiar with, such as physics or critical analysis and reasoning. While you may be able to streamline your studies and save funds for resources more urgently needed, purchasing complete sets can have advantages. First, the value of each individual book usually ends up at a discounted value compared to buying them individually. Second, since all the books are written by the same writers, they often refer to other chapters in other books, and this may help you consolidate information as you progress through your studies. Finally, purchasing complete sets usually comes with additional content that buying individually lacks, including subscriptions to online resources, concept maps, and full-length exams.

Aside from what we may call baseline preparation, there are also advanced books, which aim to prepare you to score generally within an elite percentile. It is important to note that these books are shorter in length and should generally not be relied upon to start your studying, but rather should be used to complement your studies once a strong foundation has been built.

Whether you buy individual books or the complete set, or opt to do neither, you need to consider what the different books offer, your budget, and your confidence level at the start of your preparation.

Other online resources

Online forums are a double-edged sword when it comes to MCAT preparation. They can be both a time sink and a source of anxiety, as well as a very helpful resource with many tips, study notes, and strategies on how to study. To stay productive while studying, one can allocate a certain amount of time every day to browse the forums and not exceed that limit. We found the online forum Reddit to be very useful when preparing for the MCAT. The platform can give you motivation when you feel like it is lacking, encouragement from other writers when you need it, and a multitude of free resources and study guides. For those who are more visual learners, YouTube videos can also be a helpful resource, with channels such as Khan Academy offering free MCAT videos that go over key concepts.

Another important source of resources to study for the MCAT is the AAMC. The AAMC offers full-length practice exams for purchase on their website. While it is not an inexpensive investment, since the AAMC administers the MCAT, these tests serve as the closest depiction of what the real exam situation will be like, in ways that other resources are often unable to provide. The AAMC practice exams utilize the same computer interface as the real exam, and the practice exam content accurately reflects that of the real exam. However, the true value of these practice exams is to use them to simulate a real eight-hour testing day. For such a long exam, it is important to build stamina, and these practice exams are great resources for mimicking a true testing situation, with the accurate order and length of the exam sections and designated breaks. Treating them like a real exam and running a mock testing day with start and end times for each test section are valuable mental preparations for the length of the MCAT. Given that the AAMC offers a limited number of these exams, make sure you stagger when you will take them, so they are written in a way that makes sense with your overall study schedule.

Pacing yourself: Wellness

It can be difficult to find the motivation to study for the MCAT on top of all of your other obligations, whether that be work, school, or research. In the summer, it can also be difficult to spend many long hours alone in a deserted library during beautiful days. It is important that you remember to take time for yourself during your MCAT studies. Both the preparation for the MCAT and the exam itself are marathons, not sprints. Beyond your knowledge, your ability to perform well on the test day depends on how well rested you are, your mental well-being, and your ability to stay calm during the MCAT.

To avoid burnout, remember to take breaks (see below), see friends, keep up with your hobbies, and take time off. The MCAT can be a very draining process, and taking time for yourself is very important. When you get closer to the exam, try to reduce your study load.

It is critical that you are in the right mindset the day of the exam. The day before should be a rest day where you take time for yourself and don't study at all.

Preparing to retake the MCAT

Prior to taking the exam, we recommend that you establish a personal cutoff score, whereby you would not retake the MCAT if you score above it. This will allow you to resist the urge to strive for perfection and retake an exam for which you already have a great score. It is important to note that many people do take the MCAT more than once, depending on how their first exam went and how competitive they feel it is for the current application cycle. If you feel that you need to take the exam again, do not be discouraged. While retaking this exam may feel tedious, it can also have distinct advantages in terms of increasing your score. As you are reviewing material you have already reviewed once, it is typically faster to relearn concepts that you may have forgotten, and you can now focus on topics you had more trouble with. Furthermore, you may now realize what study resources helped you prepare for the exam the first time and which did not. This enables you to adapt your studying accordingly, which can streamline your preparation. Finally, having previously taken the MCAT, you are now familiar with the process, and this may help ease some stress when you retake the exam.

DURING THE EXAM

Taking breaks

The MCAT offers three breaks. At the time of writing this book, the breaks include: a 10-minute break after each section, with a thirty-minute lunch break in the middle, for a total of three breaks (10-30-10). Different exam-taking styles will affect whether you take these breaks. Some students may decide to take the exam in one go, opting to skip all three optional breaks. Others may opt to use the breaks to refuel with drinks and snacks, a light lunch, and a short walk after sitting for an extended period. It is recommended to take breaks, as this gives some time to de-stress and take a quick breather before the next session.

Voiding your test

At the very end of the MCAT, you will be given the option to void your exam. If you choose to do so, your exam will not be scored, counted, or sent to schools—essentially there will be no record of you taking this exam. You may be wondering why you would choose to do so, after having spent the last six-plus hours taking this test. Some individuals may choose to void their exam if they felt that this testing experience did not accurately reflect their knowledge and abilities—perhaps due to feeling they had an "off day." However, just because this voiding option exists and you may not be feeling confident after the exam does not mean the decision should be made hastily. Choosing whether or not to void your exam requires some external research as well as a lot of introspection.

Prior to taking the test, it is important to look into the schools to which you are applying to see if they have any rules for how they deal with applicants that have submitted multiple MCAT exams. Some schools will take your best exam, and some will always take your most recent exam. This information is usually made public on the school's application pages. Additionally, you should be aware of the AAMC limitations on taking the MCAT multiple times in a certain period. This information is readily available on the AAMC website and may contribute to your decision on whether or not to void your exam.

Most importantly, however, is your emotional assessment of how the exam went. During your MCAT preparation, it is important to be aware of how you feel after every practice exam and to correlate that with your score. It is common to find yourself lacking confidence after every exam, even if the score turns out fine—it is possible that you only remember the questions you were stuck on (and therefore mulled over for a long time!) rather than the ones you answered right away and never looked back on. If you find yourself doing this, make a note of it and be aware that your opinion of how the real exam goes may be skewed. It may be worthwhile to make it a goal to not void your exam on the real testing day, even if you feel that now-familiar post-exam lack of confidence. This is yet another reason there is value in taking practice tests, as they provided a gauge of post-exam emotions that is useful on the actual exam day.

Nondisclosure

It is important to recall that prior to taking the MCAT, you agreed to abide by a nondisclosure agreement. It is a professional obligation to abide by this rule. As the first standardized exam of your medical career, maintaining professionalism and integrity for this exam at all stages—prior, during, and after taking it—is paramount. It ensures the integrity of this standardized exam for the medical school admission process, and it will dictate the habits with which you conduct yourself as you further your medical training.

AFTER YOU TAKE THE MCAT

Whether you feel like you scored in the ninety-ninth percentile or the first percentile, it will be very difficult for you to predict what your score is, as your feelings after the exam may not accurately reflect how you did. Furthermore, your percentile ranking depends on how everyone who took the same exam as you performed. The waiting time can be very frustrating, but remember that you gave it your all and that no matter how many times you check online premedical forums, your grade won't change. Your hard work studying for countless hours has culminated in completion of the exam. Congratulations! Finally, don't forget to take some time off for yourself; you've earned it.

CONCLUSION

In this section, we provided some background and suggestions for how we prepared for the MCAT. We have covered the first standardized test, which serves as a prerequisite for your admission to medical school. Additionally, it is important to acknowledge that the structure and content of the MCAT might change in the years following publication of this book, so your study strategies may need to be modified over time. We will now shift focus to the second important exam for many medical schools, the CASPer.

5

Standardized Testing—The CASPer

Matthew Hintermayer • Sarah Lépine • Owen Chen

Matthew Hintermayer *is a first-year MD-PhD student at McGill University. He completed his undergraduate degree in psychology at the University of Waterloo and his master's degree in Pathology and Laboratory Medicine at Western University, studying traumatic brain injury and the frontotemporal spectrum disorders associated with amyotrophic lateral sclerosis (ALS). He is currently conducting research investigating the regeneration of damaged neurons at the Montreal Neurological Institute.*

Sarah Lépine *is a second-year MD-PhD student at McGill University. She started her training in the laboratory studies program of the CEGEP of Saint-Hyacinthe and then completed an undergraduate degree in cellular and molecular biology at the University of Sherbrooke. She recently began her doctoral studies in neuroscience, and her thesis involves using stem-cell–derived culture systems to model ALS.*

Owen Chen *is a first-year MD-PhD student at McGill University. Prior to medical school, he completed both his bachelor and master of science degrees in biochemistry at McGill. He is currently pursuing his research at McGill's Goodman Cancer Research Centre, where he studies cell cycle dysregulation in cancer.*

INTRODUCTION

Historically, the Medical College Admissions Test (MCAT) was the only required standardized test when submitting applications to Canadian and American medical schools. However, in recent years medical schools have placed a larger emphasis on the nonacademic qualities of applicants that better predict those who will make good doctors. Typically, these assessments

WHAT YOU NEED TO KNOW

- The CASPer is a computerized test required for admission to some medical schools that assess nonacademic qualities.
- You can prepare for the CASPer by learning about medical ethics, problem-solving strategies, and reflecting on your personal and professional experiences dealing with conflicts.
- Questions on the CASPer can be scenario-based or resume types, each requiring a unique strategy to answer effectively and concisely.
- There are some technical considerations that you will need to take into account to succeed on the CASPer, including typing speed, time management, and the testing environment.
- Effective preparation for the CASPer involves reflecting on your skills and implementing them in your study strategy.

have been done by implementing problem-solving activities in the interview process, which assess applicants' approaches to ethical dilemmas. Some medical schools have also started using the Computer-based Assessment for Sampling Personal Characteristics (CASPer) as a standardized assessment of these "soft" skills, with results on this test comprising up to a third of an applicant's preinterview score. This current chapter will focus on the unique challenges of this intimidating and elusive test, as well as describing some general recommendations for preparation.

COMPUTER-BASED ASSESSMENT FOR SAMPLING PERSONAL CHARACTERISTICS (CASPer)

WHAT IS THE CASPer?

The CASPer is a computer-based situational judgment test designed to assess nonacademic or soft skills. Unlike the MCAT (discussed in the previous chapter), the CASPer does not require any specific content knowledge to be completed successfully. This is because, fundamentally, the CASPer is an assessment of an applicant's ability to apply logic, compassion, empathy, and critical thinking simultaneously to solve an ethical dilemma. The format and types of questions asked on the CASPer are arguably quite similar to those found in the medical school Multiple Mini Interview (MMI) format, and many schools have used this test as a way of predicting and selecting those applicants who will ultimately succeed at the interview and in clerkship during medical school. Therefore, we anticipate that the CASPer will become a more frequent component of the medical school application process in the future. In this chapter, we will further elaborate on the CASPer, illustrate why you should care about it, and share our experiences and insights on how to best approach this elusive assessment.

WHAT IS THE FORMAT OF THE CASPer?

The CASPer is taken on your home computer or laptop in a location of your choosing, while being monitored by a proctor via your computer's webcam. During the test, you are provided with twelve timed prompts that can be of two types of "setups": scenario or resume. The typical distribution of setups includes eight scenarios and four resume prompts.

The scenario-based setups might involve video clips in which you are shown an interaction displaying some sort of interpersonal or professional conflict, or they might take the format of a written prompt asking you to consider a specific topic or dilemma. Each setup is followed by three questions for which you have a total of five minutes to type your answers. After five minutes, the test automatically continues to the next question, with no ability to return to previous questions. Resume-type questions typically take the form of text prompts that ask you to think about a past experience or conflict you have had and how you handled it. Halfway through the test, you have the opportunity to take a 15-minute break to rest your eyes, drink some water, and eat a snack before beginning the second half. In total, the test is approximately 90 minutes in duration. Once you have completed the test, your answers to each of the 12 prompts are scored by 12 separate raters, and your overall score is sent directly to the medical schools you are applying to. Information regarding how answers are scored is not openly disclosed, and applicants are never informed of their CASPer scores.

PREPARING FOR THE CASPer

It is commonly stated on many Internet forums that you can't prepare for the CASPer—the rationale being that it is a test that assesses the soft skills that you cannot just study for like you would for a biochemistry exam. Indeed, the CASPer requires applicants to ponder ethical predicaments (that are not necessarily specific to medicine) and come up with possible solutions within a very restrictive time limit. The goal of this fast-paced exercise is to have candidates think on their feet and showcase social skills that take years to build. In addition, each CASPer throws in a couple of open-ended questions that require reflection of personal experiences, also a product of personal growth over many years. Taking all of this into consideration, it would make sense that preparing for this exam overnight is not possible. But from our personal experiences with taking the CASPer, we are confident that some preparation can be done to allow yourself to be more comfortable and confident on test day.

Learn principles of medical ethics and how to apply them to real-life situations

The CASPer is designed to assess your ability to make ethical decisions in difficult situations. Some key principles of medical ethics to familiarize yourself with include, but are not limited to, consent, confidentiality, disclosure, patient autonomy, and conflict of interest. You can learn more about these principles by reading books that focus on these topics. We found the book *Doing Right* by Philip C. Hébert, Oxford University Press, 1996 very useful in this regard. Keep in mind that in CASPer and medicine (and in life), there are many ethical dilemmas you will face for which there is no definitive right or wrong answer. Get more comfortable with this uncertainty by familiarizing yourself with the ways that ethicists and physicians approach these problems academically and professionally.

Know basic conflict resolution techniques

The CASPer asks many questions involving an interpersonal or professional conflict that you have to deal with. Sometimes you can be personally involved in the conflict, and you have to demonstrate how you would react in this situation. Other times, you may be asked to take on the role of a mediator and try to find some kind of compromise that suits both parties. In both cases, it often comes down to showing that you can analyze all aspects of the problem and that you have good communication skills. Some general principles of conflict management and resolution that we have found useful for the CASPer (and for life) are: de-escalation (trying to cool down the situation), choosing the right moment and the right setting to intervene, using appropriate language, encouraging dialogue, and demonstrating openness to the perspectives of others.

Reflect on your personal experiences and professional skills

The objective of the CASPer is to examine whether you possess essential competencies and skills that will make you a good doctor. Some examples of key professional abilities include leadership, communication, teamwork, professionalism, judgment, integrity, intellectual curiosity, problem solving, and dealing with stressful situations. It is important to identify what life experiences or challenges you have faced that demonstrate your possession of these skills. Before taking the test, think of concrete examples of times when you had a conflict at work or school, and how you approached resolving it. For example, think of a time when you were faced with an ethical dilemma or witnessed a lack of professionalism in a superior. What did you do, and what would you do differently should this situation arise again? On the day of the exam, you won't have time to think—you will barely have enough time to type your answers—so make sure that you have prepared concise summaries of a few key personal experiences demonstrating multiple professional skills.

Practice, practice, practice!

The CASPer is a difficult test to master, as it requires you to synthesize thoughtful responses to complex questions in a very time-constrained format. As such, the best way to develop the skills necessary for success on the CASPer is to practice answering questions in the format in which the test is written. This means obtaining questions similar to those on the CASPer and time-restricting your responses. There are many free sample questions for the CASPer available online, including a few sample questions on the CASPer website. When preparing, we put together some practice questions modified from some scenario-based MMI questions and then shared them in groups with our friends who did the same. Answering many questions in a timed setting and then reviewing your responses will help you to identify your weaknesses and how to improve on them. You may also be able to identify bad habits that can sabotage your exam. One common habit that we needed to train out of was jumping right into our decisions to ethical dilemmas before outlining the basic problem. There is more discussion of how to organize your responses to specific questions in the following section.

The general principles above should aid in your preparation of the CASPer and will likely also serve you well when preparing for the medical school interview process. In the next section, we will outline specific structuring of responses and strategies that we have used to approach answering the different question types on the CASPer.

ANSWERING QUESTIONS ON THE CASPer

As previously mentioned, there are two main types of questions you will get on the CASPer: scenario-based questions, and resume or open-ended–type questions. The ways that these questions are set up and your approach to them will likely be quite different. Although the methods that will lead you to success on the CASPer depend on your unique strengths, we have outlined some general strategies that we found useful when approaching these questions.

Scenario-based questions

These questions make up the bulk of the CASPer. Each video or text prompt presents an ethical dilemma and asks what you would do in that situation. Often, they will ask you to take a side. What can make answering these questions hard is that sometimes there is no obvious side to take. But this is completely fine! You do not need to come up with a miraculous solution in which every conflict is resolved and everyone is happy. In fact, what may be more important is that you are able to demonstrate your understanding of the conflict.

What we found helpful when answering scenario-based questions was breaking the situation down and approaching it from multiple angles and perspectives to get a better understanding of it. We did this by trying to outline the people directly and indirectly involved, the problem faced in the dilemma, and the perspectives of those in conflict. When you ultimately state your decision of what to do, consider the different outcomes and consequences of your solution and state why your decision is justified. When you outline your response in this way, the evaluator of this particular scenario will be able to see your thought process and will know that whatever your solution, you took the time to meticulously reflect on different perspectives. Do you feel you have too many thoughts to stay organized with your response? Do not worry; use the three sub-questions for each scenario as guides to write down your thought processes when coming to a decision.

Resume/open-ended questions

Resume questions, also known as open-ended questions, can take two forms: personal experience, and interpretation or personal opinion. For personal experience questions, we like to use the "STAR" method when thinking about our responses. Let's take the example of a time when you had to work with somebody difficult:

S – Situation. Come up with an anecdote where you had to work with that difficult person. Make sure you provide a bit of context to set up your response on how you managed the situation. Identify the who, what, when, where, and how.

T – Task or target. What exactly was the goal while working with that difficult person?

A – Action. What did you do to accomplish your task? How did you work with that difficult person to achieve your goal?

R – Result. Did you achieve that task with the difficult person? Did everything work out in the end? If not, why? Make sure you think about what you learned. Also, think about how you can use what you learned from this experience and apply it to similar future experiences.

As you can see from the example above, open-ended questions closely resemble traditional job interview questions. Therefore, a good way to prepare for these questions would be to re-familiarize yourself with your CV or your activities entries on your medical school applications. Think of meaningful lessons learned from each of your activities. If you forget the STAR method while taking the test, keep in mind that like the video-based scenarios, each open-ended question comes with three sub-questions, which conveniently guide you as you formulate your response to the main question. Therefore, if you have thought about STAR for your experiences during your preparation but forget to use it on the test, you should still do fine by answering the sub-questions.

You may come to see that CASPer questions resemble MMI questions in many ways. That is because schools that use the MMI format for interviews try to look for essentially the same qualities as the evaluators of the CASPer: situational judgment and soft skills that one would need to succeed as a medical professional. Therefore, you are effectively preparing for your medical school interviews as you prepare for and take the CASPer.

TECHNICAL CONSIDERATIONS FOR TAKING THE CASPer

The unique format of the CASPer test means that you must adapt your study and practice strategies to best prepare for it. As such, there are some additional technical considerations that may be overlooked by some students.

Improve your typing speed

One thing that may actually make the CASPer harder than an interview is that you are required to type your responses out, which for many people occurs at a rate much slower than talking. If you type using two to three fingers, you will likely need to improve your typing speed to do well on this test. When one of us began practicing for the CASPer, our typing rate was about 40 words per minute. This student was able to get their speed up to 70 words per minute, which was sufficient for their responses to the test. There are many websites available to assess your typing speed, and it might be useful to practice using one of these to get an understanding of where you fall. It is also worth mentioning, however, that when answering the questions on the CASPer, it is more important to get your ideas on the page quickly than to worry about proper spelling and grammar. Information on the CASPer website is very explicit in stating that you will not be penalized for spelling or grammatical errors so long as your ideas are clear. We are aware of one instance where a student spelled the word "interdisciplinary" with an "*" instead of an "i" and was still successful regardless.

Have a reliable Internet connection

This point seems like common sense but is important enough to state explicitly. Ensuring that you have a reliable Internet connection is essential to your success during the CASPer. The test goes by very quickly, and a lagging Internet connection might hijack valuable seconds that you could be using to type your responses. Do not let a slow Internet connection be the reason your application is not viewed favorably. If the Internet in your home is slow, take the test in a space with a reliable connection. Although your answers will be saved and you will not lose test time in the event of a disconnection (or power loss), a reliable Internet connection can reduce a lot of stress on test day.

Avoid stimulating environments

We imagine that most people reading this book will have experience with taking exams, so this shouldn't be a shock to anyone. The CASPer requires you to focus, as you will be watching videos of interactions in real time without the ability to watch them again or rewind. As such, you will need to be focused so that you can pick out important information from the video prompts. Wear earphones instead of playing the sounds through your speakers, to limit the blending of sounds in your environment with those in the video. Do the test in a cubicle or an even less stimulating location to avoid visual distractions.

Schedule more time on test day than you think you will need

As with any online test with a large number of individuals taking it simultaneously, there is a certain amount of technical error that can occur. Although the company responsible for the CASPer does an excellent job at maintaining their server strength for test day, there is still the possibility that your test will be delayed. You should not expect a delay, but be prepared for one. For one of the times we took the test, our time slots were pushed back a few hours due to technical difficulties, and one of us needed to call into their workplace to let them know they could not come in for their shift. We recommend keeping a couple of hours free after the test just in case there are technical problems. Besides, this test is tiring, and you may benefit from taking a break after it should your test run as scheduled.

HOW MANY TIMES DO I NEED TO COMPLETE THE CASPer?

There are at least three variables that will determine how many times you will need to complete the CASPer. First, are you applying to other professional programs that require the CASPer? Second, are you applying to schools that require different CASPer tests? Third, how many application cycles will you go through before you are successful in getting into medical school?

Many of us needed to keep our options open when we decided that a career in health care was where we belonged. We all applied to many medical schools. Some of us applied numerous times and eventually were successful in matriculating at McGill University. However, to keep their options open, one of us also applied to nursing school to ensure that they had other ways of pursuing a career in health care in the event that they were not successful in getting into medical school. Indeed, when they applied to nursing school, they needed to take a different CASPer than the one that they had written for their medical school application that year. That meant paying extra fees, getting an extra day off work, and going through all of the preparation twice. Different CASPer questions are asked depending on the program you are applying to, and the answers may even be assessed in different ways and on different parameters. This is important to consider if you are applying to other professional schools that require a different version of the CASPer. If you are unsure, it is best to contact the admissions department to verify these details.

Additionally, some schools may even have different CASPer requirements. This means that even if you are only applying to medical schools in North America, you may still need to complete the CASPer more than once in a given application cycle to satisfy the requirements of each school. Again, this is something that you should look into prior to submitting the first parts of your application to these schools, if the cost of taking the CASPer is significant to you. If it is unclear whether or not a given school will accept the particular version of the CASPer test you are taking (i.e., the specific testing date), verify with the school.

Finally, unlike the MCAT (for which scores are typically valid for a period of 3–5 years, depending on the medical school), your results on the CASPer are typically only valid for a single application cycle. This means that if you apply 1 year and are not successful in matriculating into medical school, you must complete the CASPer again the next time you apply. We are aware of at least one individual who was applying to medical school for a second time and had assumed he did not need to take the CASPer again. He did end up taking the test in time, but this misconception almost cost him any chance of getting into any medical school for which the CASPer was required.

CONCLUSION

In this chapter we have introduced you to the CASPer, a standardized assessment of your nonacademic qualities. We have outlined why it is important to prepare for the CASPer and have given you some useful suggestions regarding how to prepare for this intimidating test. Ultimately, the decision of how to prepare for this test will depend on your own strengths and weaknesses, so we encourage you to personalize how you implement our suggestions while you prepare. Additionally, it is important to acknowledge that the structure and content of the CASPer might change in the years following publication of this book. The general recommendations stated in this chapter should still apply and be useful to you, but the specific ways in which these recommendations are implemented may need to be modified with changes to the CASPer in mind. Best of luck.

6

Building Your MD-PhD Application

Mack A. Michell-Robinson

Mack A. Michell-Robinson *is a third-year MD-PhD student at McGill University. His PhD research is in the field of neurology, focusing on developing experimental models of a rare disease of the central nervous system, along with gene therapies to treat it. Prior to medical school, Mack completed both bachelor and master of science degrees at McGill University, and worked as an associate scientist at a Fortune 500 biotechnology company.*

INTRODUCTION

This chapter and Chapter 7 ("The Application Process and the Interviews") complement one another, and both contain important advice that contribute to creating the best final application possible, divided loosely according to the typical chronological order. In this chapter, we'll consider the building blocks of successful applications as you assemble them in the last few months before you plan to apply. An MD-PhD application is essentially an MD application with a specific research focus. Therefore, this chapter necessarily covers the building blocks of the MD application from the perspective of what an MD-PhD committee will be looking for. Specifically, we will cover the basics of admissions, standardized testing, grades, how to build research experiences and communicate research potential, publications and presentations, volunteering and humanitarianism, work experiences, extracurricular

> **WHAT YOU NEED TO KNOW**
>
> - Deadlines, especially for expiration of standardized tests like the MCAT, vary by institution. Make a spreadsheet of important deadlines and set calendar reminders!
> - Academic excellence, especially grades, is the most important part of the medical school admissions process. Meanwhile, showing your commitment to research is the most important part of the PhD admissions process.
> - Jobs, extracurricular activities, and volunteering provide necessary life experiences that make you a more interesting candidate (and hopefully a more interesting person!).
> - When writing your personal statement, keep it simple, authentic, and reflective. Ask yourself: "How can I have the greatest impact, and why do I want to?"
> - When writing your research statement, stay on message, and focus on the impact of your work. Answer the question: "Why is this important?"

involvement, and writing essays, statements, and narratives with a focus on writing research statements. It is recommended that you reread Chapter 2 ("Choosing the Right MD-PhD Program for You") and have schools in mind while building your application so that you know where to concentrate your time and effort. Each application is unique to the applicant; this chapter will describe what you'll be expected to include to be considered competitive, with specific insights for MD-PhD aspirants.

ADMISSIONS BASICS

Using guidelines to write an application

When assembling an application, it is essential to read the admissions handbook, the guidelines, or any other published admissions materials (statistics, etc.) for the program you're applying to. Sometimes, they'll have different names, but they can usually be found on a corresponding MD program's website. This is critical to the application-building process, because each program will use different weighing systems when ranking applicants. In fact, while the building blocks composing applications are similar between medical schools, two different medical schools often rank an identical pool of applications quite differently. Any available statistics and guidelines should be used to fit the building blocks discussed in the chapter into your final application in the way the program expects. While having amazing scores, grades, and experiences is a great asset, these guidelines must be observed so that your application ranks as highly as possible.

How medical schools handle applications

The admissions process, that is, what happens after you submit your application to a program, is highly variable between medical schools. However, there are some generalities to understand when reading the rest of the chapter. In the first round of applications, applicants will be triaged; those who meet numerical cutoff values and/or other minimum requirements such as prerequisites move forward in the process. Some programs may evaluate all applications without triaging first, but the result is the same.

Candidate applications that meet minimum requirements will then be scored and ranked according to the internal guidelines set by the institution. Applicants who rank above a threshold will be invited for the second round of applications, which usually involves interviews (Chapter 7). Following the second round of applications, students will again be scored and ranked on the basis of interview performance according to internal guidelines. The second round of applications at some schools may use a composite scoring system involving the applicant's grades or other application materials from round one.

Finally, the program will rank applicants on their performance in rounds one and two and invite successful applicants to reserve a position in the class for the upcoming year. As this process varies widely by program, I would like to reiterate the importance of reading and understanding the admissions guidelines or handbook for the program you wish to apply for while building your application. The following sections will concentrate on the individual elements that make up your applicant profile, each contributing to your application's rank.

STANDARDIZED TESTING

Standardized testing is a necessary element for application to many medical schools. In the United States and many institutions in Canada, the Medical College Admission Test (MCAT) is the required standardized test. There are a few graduate faculties that require the

Graduate Management Admission Test (GMAT) or Graduate Record Examination (GRE) as part of their PhD admission requirement, and you may be required to write one of these as well, although this is less common for MD-PhD programs. Therefore, it will be necessary to know well in advance whether you will need to have written one or more standardized tests when building an MD-PhD application. To this end, it is important to consider how medical schools consider your scores, as well as any deadlines and expiration dates involved (see below). Chapter 4 ("Standardized Testing—The MCAT") and Chapter 5 ("Standardized Testing—The CASPer") can be reviewed if you are doing either of those tests.

Ranking test scores and numerical ranges

Numerical ranges for MCAT testing results from matriculated students will commonly be published on a medical school website or in an admissions handbook and should be consulted in advance of writing the test or applying. Each school will use these scores differently; minimally, they will be used as a numerical cutoff where a minimum score is required to advance the application to the second round. Oftentimes, your score will be factored into the overall ranking of your application, and to this end, different sections of the exam may be weighted individually. These weights and values may influence your approach to writing the exam and will be critical when considering whether your scores will be competitive.

ACADEMIC TRACK RECORD

The academic track record (your grades) you build during your basis-of-admission degree is one of the most important parts of your application. The basis-of-admission degree is usually an undergraduate degree; however, some schools may calculate a composite score based on more than one degree (see below). A good academic track record will be important for the preinterview application round, and some components of the track record can also be critical in subsequent rounds of admission, depending on the institution. Look at the admissions statistics for the institutions you plan on applying to in order to see if your grades fit the profile of applicants who matriculate. Looking at this type of data can also help inform the development of your application for a given school, because if you consult it well in advance (e.g., during your basis-of-admission degree), you can tailor your efforts to match the requirements at your institution of choice. Bear in mind that prerequisite courses, especially science ones, may be considered separately in some programs. For example, a school may require a minimum 3.6/4.0 cumulative grade point average (GPA), but also require meeting a GPA cutoff for prerequisite science credits (biology, chemistry, etc.). These facts are laid out in the admission guidelines of each institution.

Performance and GPA

The academic track record of an applicant will be evaluated to ascertain whether a candidate has achieved the cutoff values and/or where they fit into the distribution of current applicants and/or previously selected candidate GPAs. Ultimately, GPA values are a major factor in ranking applicants relative to one another. A better GPA is always preferable, and readers who are undergraduates should strive to achieve the highest grades possible. It is safe to say that the number of applicants at any mid- to large-size institution in North America will virtually guarantee that, statistically speaking, the distribution of GPAs across an applicant pool is unlikely to differ much from one year to another. Therefore, if your basis-of-admission GPA is already established, falls within the distribution of previously selected GPAs, and you did not interview after submitting an application, your best option for a subsequent application is working on the other aspects of your profile. You may decide to pursue further education such as graduate training if your GPA is near the lower end of the distribution (see below). High performance during the undergraduate degree will expedite the process of building an application more than any other aspect of your profile.

How to build an academic track record to support an MD-PhD application

After high school, students in the United States or Canada usually complete an undergraduate degree before applying to medical school. The undergraduate degree should generally be in life sciences (biology, health sciences, anatomy, physiology, etc.) to allow you to complete the science prerequisites for most programs. However, other applicants may take a math, physics, engineering, or arts/humanities-based undergraduate degree and complete their life science prerequisites in addition. An arts-based undergraduate degree will require near-perfect grades to achieve, as non-science undergraduate tracks will be scrutinized more heavily to ensure compliance with institutional prerequisites, and arts/humanities course loads may be perceived as less intense than other areas of study. Overall, it is advisable to pick an undergraduate track at an institution that will provide a well-respected degree at the conclusion of your studies and allow you to meet medical school prerequisites.

Where scheduling is concerned, make sure to take a full course load each semester and avoid overloading an individual semester with heavy courses to give you the best chance of success across all the courses you take. Cumulative GPA cutoffs will vary across medical programs, so there are two approaches to grade goal setting: either aim to ace everything you take or strategize and plan your scheduling meticulously to excel in the most important courses. Preparatory courses similar to those for studying for the MCAT are often available to students for courses such as introductory biology, chemistry, physics, and/or calculus. These are highly recommended in order to guarantee results, especially in subjects that you consider a personal weakness. It is important to take your GPA seriously when planning to apply for an MD-PhD training program, as the results you obtain in your undergraduate program are most often used for the basis-of-admission degree.

What to do if your undergraduate degree was less than perfect

After completing an undergraduate degree with a less competitive GPA, you may choose to pursue a graduate degree (MS or PhD) before applying to an MD-PhD program. Some students may have the option of pursuing a second undergraduate degree, although this is less common. Another option is called a Special Master's Program (SMP) which is a 1- to 2-year postbaccalaureate training program focused on enhancing premedical students' academic records. These programs are costly, but they allow students to take premedical coursework specifically geared to meet medical school prerequisites, and they train students to succeed on the MCAT. SMPs are gaining traction in the United States, are offered at many major institutions, and may represent a viable option where GPA is a problem and funding circumstances permit. Because the coursework is geared toward meeting medical school prerequisite credits, these courses can help improve your GPA as calculated by the program of your choice.

However, keep in mind that you should always check the guidelines at the institution you hope to attend in order to determine how these postbaccalaureate credits will be treated in calculating your basis-of-admission grades. If your target medical school does not consider these grades as part of the basis of admission, you may decide to pursue a graduate degree (usually an MS). The advantages of pursuing a graduate degree include additional opportunities to enhance your GPA as well as establishing other application profile aspects, including research experiences, publications, and presentations that are invaluable to MD-PhD applicants.

Applying to MD-PhD programs with more than one degree

Some individuals will apply to medical school from various levels of graduate training. For these students, understanding how a medical school will assess their basis-of-admission grades is crucial. For instance, some schools will consider an MS GPA to be worth 1–2 years of full-time equivalent undergraduate coursework. Others will not consider the MS GPA as relevant whatsoever. Some schools will put applicants with a prior MS or PhD in a different applicant pool entirely. Most schools will still rely on undergraduate prerequisite courses for some part of the basis-of-admission GPA calculation. These kinds of assessments can change the application landscape completely from one institution to the next, so pick your targets wisely. If GPA is not an issue but you have completed graduate training, your graduate training will likely help your application stand out to an MD-PhD admissions committee. Finally, if you are considering entering an MD-PhD program from a graduate program and the guidebook is inconclusive with respect to GPA calculations for the basis of admission, it may be worthwhile meeting with an admissions representative for the program to determine how you would be evaluated in their admissions process.

RESEARCH EXPERIENCE

Most MD-PhD programs provide a mechanism for pursuing a PhD in almost any field. However, the vast majority of students pursue biomedical research. In that context, we will begin with aspects of building the research profile, because it is a critically important part of both the MD and PhD application. After all, MD-PhD programs are searching for candidates who will make excellent future researchers. A cornerstone of MD-PhD education is producing graduates with the ability to do inspired work in the science, technology, engineering, and math (STEM) fields; succeed at obtaining grant funding; and participate in communicating novel results via publications and conferences. The MD portion of an application will not demand such a high level of commitment to science, but applying to an MD-PhD program will guarantee both a higher level of competition and critique from the PhD applications committee. Therefore, it serves well in both the MD and PhD application to spend significant time building this aspect of your profile.

How to build research experiences through volunteer and paid lab work

To demonstrate research commitment, students should strive to participate in research activities, especially laboratory work experiences. Semester-long research seminars and lab rotations are fine, but for any medical school applicant with MD-PhD aspirations, a major aim of any research activities should be to build fundamental research skills and participate in publishing a manuscript or presenting findings in a public forum. These are also the major avenues for graduate students to participate in the larger scientific community and represent an essential aspect of being an academic scientist. If you are early enough in your bachelor's degree (e.g., first year), consider declaring an honors-program major with a year or more research component that could provide access to a lab and/or project.

Otherwise, summer research as a bachelor's student can also show initiative and may produce an academic network that facilitates publications. Other avenues to consider include writing letters to the editor about recent publications or reviews for postdoctoral students/ academic staff while working or volunteering in a lab. These all demonstrate serious consideration and knowledge of a scientific field as well as an ability to write effectively. Since writing for publication in an academic field can be an exacting process for the uninitiated, it helps to have an allied postdoctoral or PhD student to guide you. In all these cases, the goal is to participate in scientific research, writing, and presentations—crucial skills required for graduate students to succeed. Always remember to get your senior colleagues' references to back up your hard work on your application.

Communicating your potential and commitment to research

In order to communicate your research potential to an application committee, you will need to have worked on one or more serious research projects. Having a master's degree (research thesis) in an STEM field or a prior job as a scientist can be incredibly beneficial in this respect, especially if you have published results to show for your efforts. In short, merely communicating that you may have skills in common with excellent researchers or that you value critical thinking will not be enough.

If you are coming from a bachelor's-degree background, it will be especially important to demonstrate commitment to research to be a competitive applicant. Since the applications committee is deciding whether to allocate a large amount of resources to your training as a scientist, they want to be convinced that you are serious about becoming a physician-researcher. If you have done significant research, think about ways to highlight your skills and experiences. It is important to be able to discuss concepts, such as aspects of your research skill set, that you want to develop further, and ways that you intend to use past experiences to inform your future work. To do so, reflect on your research profile as a stranger would and reacquaint yourself with past work. Sometimes it helps to write a paragraph describing what a study you worked on means and why it is important, as though you were writing for a layperson. Consider the strengths and weaknesses of your work and how you might address them through skill development.

Get your references from past supervisors in order as early as possible; although glowing references are always best, a simple confirmation of your participation in research activities and the extent of your participation will suffice in some cases. It is common to provide a list or rough draft detailing your research activities to a former supervisor when asking for a reference, for the supervisor's convenience. Communicating your research potential is a critical exercise and should be practiced before it comes time to write your application.

Publications and presentations

Your goal in building a research profile for applying to an MD-PhD program is to demonstrate that you are a committed candidate with a serious research background for your level. While authorship of novel work in a published manuscript on your CV is considered to be the best way to demonstrate this, it is recognized that some labs (and some fields, more generally) do not publish as frequently as others. Therefore, contributions in the form of letters and reviews are also highly valued. Finally, working for a well-known researcher or lab/institute is important, since a well-known entity will always outrank a lesser-known one in applications, regardless of the quality of the work. This reality is harsh but speaks to the time constraints imposed on any review committee—an established track record always prevails.

If you have the opportunity to collaborate with a researcher at the institution you intend to apply to, this is highly recommended, as this name is more likely to be known at their home university. Manuscripts submitted for publication are considered equal to published ones by many medical schools when evaluating candidates. However, be aware that the PhD evaluation committee may feel more strongly in favor of candidates with more established publication records, and yours will likely be evaluated against the competition within your applicant pool.

Communicating nontraditional contributions to laboratory research is always recommended; for instance, specific contributions to setting up assays, experiments, or data analysis techniques can be a good way to show research proficiency regardless of your publication status. Finally, scientific communications such as posters, abstracts, presentations, and talks are all great ways to demonstrate communication with the scientific public that are invaluable to an MD-PhD applicant.

VOLUNTEERING AND HUMANITARIANISM

Volunteering has always been a cornerstone of the medical school application. Medicine relies on students and residents to perform a large number of duties that can be difficult, at times unreasonably so, all in the interest of the public good. Therefore, it is important to demonstrate that you are a motivated altruist with public service at heart. An old adage refers to "three hundred hours" of requisite volunteering for candidacy in a medical program. I am not aware of a true numerical cutoff, although it may exist in some programs.

When considering the volunteering aspect of an applicant profile, keep in mind that demonstrating a track record of humanitarianism is most important. A track record of volunteering over multiple years, as far back as possible, is highly beneficial, as it demonstrates continuity and commitment to a cause. For instance, volunteering one to three hours per week with senior citizens over several years can demonstrate significant impact in a community. Furthermore, a diversity of projects can demonstrate a true altruistic interest in others; try volunteering in several different projects of variable length, with different populations. Finally, make sure that at least one of your volunteering experiences places you in a facility directly responsible for health care. Whether this is a senior care facility or a hospital, it is a genuine opportunity to demonstrate a commitment to health care and gives you the opportunity to truly consider your decision to work in clinical practice.

For those with a less significant volunteering background and little time to build one, much emphasis has been put on "voluntourism." Spending several weeks on a large volunteering excursion in a foreign country to help with public health projects—for instance, building wells or delivering medical supplies—is a common way for students to augment their volunteering. However, it can be incredibly expensive and is by no means the only way to build the humanitarian aspect of your applicant profile—a track record of volunteering is more important than one big trip. Voluntourism is also increasingly controversial. The immediate results of work like this can have astounding short-term positive impact in some places. However, experts have begun to be more critical of this approach and whether it may actually be detrimental to local residents over the longer term. Therefore, it will be important to carefully choose a project by considering its longevity, how it will impact residents in 5 or even 10 years, how the group you're working for manages to collaborate with other groups in the region, and the capacity of the group you're working with to empower local allies. Being prepared to discuss these aspects of your volunteering trip in essay or interview format will demonstrate thoughtfulness and attention to detail, as well as familiarity with a modern public health issue that involves medical students.

WORK EXPERIENCES

Work experiences are a key part of the medical school application because they communicate life experience and demonstrate certain aspects of maturity that cannot be learned in other ways. An admissions committee will be looking for a candidate with enough life experience to make the decision to study medicine, which is considered by almost all doctors to be a lifelong journey. Furthermore, medicine is a career—it shouldn't be your first job.

There are probably no hard rules for deciding what work experiences are best in a medical application. If you have the opportunity to pick a work experience with a public service or medical aspect, it could be beneficial to do so. However, having a diversity of experiences in your past is a component of the work experience profile that also demonstrates maturity. Try to take hold of diverse opportunities in your work experiences, because they all have unique advantages and lessons to be learned. However, if you plan on working during school, try to limit your number of hours, so that it does not affect the outcome of your grades, which are ultimately more important for your application.

EXTRACURRICULAR ACTIVITIES

Extracurricular activities are a part of the medical school application process that helps you demonstrate participation in your community of peers. In short, how will you contribute to your medical class community? Extracurricular activities include sports (varsity, intramural), student government and associations, music, and social or other interest groups at your university. Although these are rarely key factors for entrance on their own, they can distinguish you as a personable candidate and give the admissions committee an idea of your capacity as a catalyst and organizer of your peers.

For MD-PhD applicants, it may be useful to join research interest groups, journal clubs, and student publishing groups. Furthermore, if you were heavily engaged in extracurricular activities during a degree, it can help offset the perception of average grades or give you an impressive boost if your grades were excellent. When writing your application, make sure to focus on how participation in extracurricular activities helped you develop transferable skills, and how this personal development will inform your path to becoming a medical doctor.

WRITING APPLICATION ESSAYS, STATEMENTS, AND THE PERSONAL NARRATIVE

When writing an essay, statement, or narrative for medical school, you must first realize they all have the same underlying requirement. Here, the all-important personal narrative must be mastered in order to convey how your experiences have been woven together to produce you, the perfect candidate. Once you know how to write your narrative, you can tailor this information to respond to the specific prompt demanded by the application. Remember that you may be asked any number of individual questions; what the reader really wants to know is who is answering it.

Ultimately, the narrative you construct will form the backbone of each of your essays in their different forms, including the research statement, specifically discussed at the end of this chapter. In order to help you with your practice, I have included a number of elements that are universally present in good responses to application prompts. It is advisable before you write your application to write several general statements that approach your experiences from different angles. You may find one or two that work better than the others, and this will help you frame your writing when you're finally working on your actual drafts.

Active voice

Demonstrate intention in your activities using the active voice in your writing: "I changed the face of medicine by helping invent a new cancer therapy" versus "the face of medicine was changed by a new cancer therapy I helped invent." The active voice is far more enjoyable and readable, but it isn't always readily at hand for candidates who are used to writing in a technical, scientific style.

Personal reflection

Demonstrate maturity and self-reflection by constructing a narrative of personal growth and achievement. Reflect on how and why you accomplished something. How did you impact that thing, and importantly, how did it impact you? Furthermore, reflect on how something you did created an impact on others around you and why this is important to you and them. Personal reflection should not be self-involved; it is simply an opportunity to reflect on the internal states that lead us in new directions. Personal reflection is an opportunity to address the larger question: "How can I have the greatest impact and why do I want to?"

Service

When answering interview questions and writing personal statements, always remember to emphasize what you can offer and how you can help, while de-emphasizing how you might personally gain knowledge, training, skills, or other benefits through involvement in an organization. It may feel impossible to benefit an organization that you have never been a part of, but everyone has something to offer, and it is vitally important to understand how you will contribute to the environment in which you will work and learn.

Overcoming obstacles

Many medical schools ask essay questions about overcoming adversity, challenges undertaken, and persistence in the face of overwhelming odds. These questions aim at understanding a candidate's experiences with difficulty, because medical school poses challenges to almost every student at some point during their education. What have you learned in the past that will help you handle yourself in the challenges to come? How have you grown? How are you better now for your hard work and personal growth?

These questions will be important to consider when you construct your personal narrative, so that you can demonstrate perseverance. Writing about scenarios where you decided to undertake a personal or professional challenge is the best way to discuss overcoming obstacles in the context of an application. Framing a discussion around personal hardships is trickier, and it can be more difficult to give the required context for an appropriate discussion within the confines of the word limit.

Straight line

If you're like me and don't have the skill set of a creative writer, make your narrative arc a straight line. Since it will be the first time the reviewer has ever heard your story, keep it as simple as possible. Pick a few of your most prized accomplishments/projects and declare them in your introduction. Use your introduction to make a point about how these events answer the prompt. Then construct a simple narrative through each of these events. Try to link them using transitional sentences that clarify and simplify the decision-making process involved in moving from one project/event to another. Whether you pick a chronological order or some other order of events (projects or jobs, for example) to describe yourself and your accomplishments, make this clear and consistent throughout your writing. This will help an overworked application reviewer understand your writing on the first read through.

Respond to the prompt

When writing applications of any kind, I often copy and paste the prompt into a Word document and answer the specific parts of the prompt in simple bullet points. Further down in the document, I will copy and paste that text into a rough outline of the essay that keeps the same form as the order of the specific points that were asked in the prompt. Here, I add opening sentences and concluding sentences around the points that aim to respond to the prompt. I also incorporate specific language and keywords from the prompt into the introductory, lead-in, or concluding sentences, which will help a reader who is merely scanning the document to identify sections where I have answered a specific part of the prompt. Then, I fill in the bullet points with my experiences and refine them. Finally, in the conclusion, I demonstrate how the points I made answer the prompt and make a final statement answering their question, which directly uses the specific terminology from the prompt. Using these tips and tricks will help you incorporate your thoughts and experiences into simple statements that will not obfuscate your response to the prompt.

Summarize and conclude

Remember that the human brain has a fixed attention span. You may well be the hundredth application reviewed by an admissions employee or volunteer. Use summarizing and concluding sentences and paragraphs to package your message and make it digestible to the overwhelmed brain. Consider using headings to separate your narrative into clear sections that are outlined in an introductory paragraph. State what you mean up front, qualify it, summarize, and conclude, linking to your next paragraph. This cannot be overemphasized, as a clear message is the most important aspect of the personal narrative—it will be read only once.

Get an editor

This is rule number one, but it isn't at the top of the list, because you must write before you can edit. The most important part of any writing endeavor is to get an editor (unless you are a best-selling author, in which case you may have one). I usually have three or four different people edit my applications, and I pick editors from different parts of my life. Some are academic, some are from other fields, and some have lay understanding of science in general. Having a trusted second or third pair of eyes looking over your application is the only way to know for sure that your message is conveyed in the most understandable way to the broadest audience. When asking for edits, ask specific questions: "What emotions does this section evoke?" "What is your first impression of this text/paragraph?" "What did you think I meant here?" This will help you get the impression you are creating in your writing, which is what a reviewer will ultimately be making their judgment on.

THE RESEARCH STATEMENT—A PROFESSIONAL NARRATIVE

The research statement is a professional narrative, not a personal one. Certain stylistic tendencies are expected. The text is more conservative in tone and places less emphasis on personal reflection and feeling. This section will discuss the structure of a research statement, its tone and voice, and your adherence to some of the narrative rules discussed in the section above.

Structure

The body of a good research statement is usually based on a chronological description of one's research activities. It is an important opportunity to discuss the impact or intention behind your work, as well as the ways in which you contributed to it. I like to discuss my motivation for my research in the opening paragraph, along with my future goal (in your case, MD-PhD studies) and how this connects to the work to be described in the statement. While describing the work in subsequent paragraphs, I think it is important to emphasize the impact of the work (publications, conferences, grants, awards) more than the technical nature of the work itself. This is because for this specific type of application, it is unlikely that your reviewer will have knowledge of your field, while the measures of research impact are the same across scientific domains.

Be sure to create clear links as you move forward in the discussion through various projects or events that have shaped you research career. Keep the line plain and apparent by demonstrating why you moved from project to project. Finally, do not make the mistake of leaving out a concluding paragraph that clearly states how you intend to further your contribution to the sciences through the MD-PhD program. When writing the conclusion, imagine you're answering a reviewer asking: "What do you want to accomplish by submitting this application?" However, throughout the research statement, you must observe certain writing conventions that are specific to scientific writing.

Tone and voice

The research statement is perhaps best understood as a narrative in which you must demonstrate the importance of your work, bending many of the rules previously stated in order to observe scientific conventions of tone and voice. I see most research statements as having an instructive or informative tone, whereas other types of statements may be more reflective and have a freer style. Despite this stylistic expectation, researchers don't always communicate well across fields, so it is important to minimize technical jargon and acronyms as much as possible.

To be conservative, I tend to employ a method where I will use a minimum of technical language to describe specific techniques or experiments, followed by a sentence describing the importance or impact of my work using lay language. You really can't afford to use more than one technical sentence at a time, or you are likely to lose the reviewer's attention. In my opinion, you should always be answering the reader's unspoken question: "Why is this important?"

Other conventions

As for how your research statement should treat the rules previously discussed for personal statements and narratives, the answers are less obvious. The active voice is less of a requirement in a research statement, but you should still try to use it as consistently as possible. Personal reflection is not necessarily a rule to break in the research statement but must be treated more conservatively. Instead of focusing on statements of opinion or feeling, lead with logic. For instance, discuss how your work on one project influenced your decision to pursue another rather than declaring an interest in it based on personal circumstance. Finally, service to a cause (other than research or a disease area itself) and overcoming (personal) obstacles don't need to be discussed unless specifically prompted. These can be powerful tools in specific cases, but for most they should probably be avoided. However, you can frame your work in terms of research obstacles such as difficult questions within your field that you were involved in tackling. The rule of thumb: don't discuss personal circumstances unless they are truly extraordinary; rather, focus on the work. Since the research statement is more of a professional letter than the personal statement, highlighting your accomplishments should be given priority.

Summary

The research statement is a modified personal narrative covering your research activities and achievements and set in the frame of your overarching goal of contributing to science. It is important to maintain a more instructive and conservative tone when writing a research statement. Observe scientific writing conventions as much as possible but keep in mind that your application is likely to be read by someone outside your field. Therefore, minimize jargon and focus on the impact of your work. It is a good idea to have a look at research statements written by others before you write your own in order to get a feel for the specific tone and writing conventions involved, especially if you haven't written one before. Remember to get an editor to look over your research statement after it is written in order to ensure that your points are made clearly and concisely.

CONCLUSION

In this chapter, we discussed building an application package using the various building blocks expected of MD-PhD applicants. These include your academic track record but also research, volunteer, work, and extracurricular experiences. We also discussed universal aspects of good personal narrative statements, which form the basis of almost every medical school essay question. A piece of advice—write your personal narrative in advance and tailor it to meet the needs of a given application; you will avoid stress and save time. Finally, I wish you the best of luck in achieving your MD-PhD goal, and I hope you enjoy the rest of the guide.

7

The Application Process and the Interviews

Dominique Geoffrion

Dominique Geoffrion *is a second-year MD-PhD student at McGill University. Her PhD research is in experimental surgery and aims at uncovering and targeting functional mediators of glaucoma development following corneal transplantation surgery in order to save patients from irreversible blindness. Prior to medical school, Dominique Geoffrion completed a bachelor of science with honors in biomedical sciences from the Université de Montréal.*

INTRODUCTION

In this chapter, the MD-PhD application process is presented, including the time line and interviews for both the MD and PhD programs. The process is lengthy, and it requires planning, time, and dedication. Nonetheless, it allows applicants to reflect on both their accomplishments and hardships. The first steps of the process, positioning yourself for a successful application and building your application, were addressed in Chapters 3 and 6, respectively. I particularly recommend you review Chapter 6. Although the advice there is aimed for students who are earlier in the process than you are, no application process

---

WHAT YOU NEED TO KNOW

- Get involved in research early on and as much as possible, aiming for diversity (papers, theses, oral presentations, poster presentations).
- Work on your application documents a lot, and ask other people to read them and give you constructive feedback about what to edit and what to value most.
- Ensure a balance for each category that is being evaluated by the university, rather than trying to be a stellar applicant in one category.
- Understand and practice the interview format used at your university of choice, as it can throw you off easily even if you are well prepared or a naturally gifted public speaker.
- Do not get discouraged if your application is not successful the first time; understand the reasons, change your application documents, and reapply every time with your head held high.

is completely linear. This chapter includes a review of the components of an application, provides my own perspective on them, and aims to create the most polished product possible for you to send in. It is crucial to be aware of not only what is expected in terms of application requirements but also of how the process unfolds throughout the months prior to admission. As a student currently in the second year of the MD, CM, and PhD program at McGill University and in the first year of my PhD, I have recently been through the application process myself. I hope to shine some light on the key elements of applying to a combined MD and PhD degree program.

THE MILESTONES OF THE APPLICATION PROCESS

Applying to a medical program can be a daunting task with many variables to consider. An application should be competitive in both the MD and the PhD applicant pools. It may require applying to each program either separately or together, depending on the university. The MD application component should not be overlooked. It can even represent the bigger challenge, given that the applicant pool is larger, and available positions in medical programs are fewer than in graduate programs.

Overview of the process

There are two stages of applying to medical school: (1) the initial application to get invited to interviews, and (2) preparing for the interviews in order to receive a final offer of admission. The first stage includes scheduling and preparing for the Medical College Admissions Test (MCAT), written and administered by the American Association of Medical Colleges (AAMC). Other tests may be required, most notably the Computer-Based Assessment for Sampling Personal Characteristics (CASPer) test, which is a part of the application process for some Canadian and American universities. Chapter 4 was dedicated to informing and preparing students for the MCAT, and Chapter 5 did the same for the CASPer.

The other components accounting for the rest of the total score may include cumulative GPA, curriculum vitae, and grades for basic science courses, to name a few. This also varies across universities. Documents for the PhD component of the application generally include a personal narrative or letter of intent, letters of reference, and a summary of previous research activities.

Overall, the complete application must be submitted for evaluation before the deadline set by the university. Transcripts from previous academic institutions must be ordered months before the deadline. Once applications are submitted, interview invitations are offered a few months later. Prospective candidates then prepare, often during approximately one month, for the second stage of the process, which is the interviews for both the MD and PhD programs. The ultimate goal is to receive an offer of admission from the desired university offering the joint MD-PhD program.

Each application must be specifically tailored to the institution and to the cycle of application of the current year. Requirements change per university and per cycle of admission. Each institution will have a precise list of documents required as part of the application, as well as an indication of what the selection committee values as skills and competencies in successful candidates. This information will be useful to the candidate to write the different application components and effectively communicate their potential for that specific institution.

In summary, there are several crucial aspects of medical school applications: standardized testing, academic excellence, research experience, volunteering, work experience, and extracurricular activities. Research experience will be particularly important when applying to a combined MD-PhD program and includes research projects, written reports and theses, poster presentations, oral presentations, scholarships, and publications in peer-reviewed journals. The different steps and application components will be explained in this chapter.

Preparing the curriculum vitae

Chapter 6 covers in depth all the components you need to collect to be ready to apply, and I suggest you review the details of that chapter. Now, you trim those components down to make the best application according to the guidelines you are given. The curriculum vitae (CV) required as part of the medical school application might be limited in terms of length or years to cover. Therefore, some applicants might need to select only a few activities and experiences from their CV, based on the skills that were learned or developed during each activity. In addition to excellent grades, the CV will aid the selection committee in understanding who you are as a person and what unique skills you have to offer. Different work, volunteering, and extracurricular experiences should reflect a wide array of leadership and social skills. These skills include autonomy, initiative, creativity, curiosity, teamwork, empathy, and communication skills. For each activity in the CV, a few details can be presented. These can include: a brief role description, a list of the qualities and skills that were acquired or developed during this activity, and a description of the lessons learned. These qualities and skills can be drawn from the university admissions instructions. Making sure to assign at least one quality to each activity mentioned in the CV ensures that the chosen activities demonstrate a wide variety of competencies that are sought after in potential candidates.

The research component of the CV will be particularly important when applying to a joint MD-PhD program. This might include research projects, written reports for undergraduate internships, graduate theses, poster presentations, oral presentations, scholarships, and publications in peer-reviewed journals. Any written report, publication, or presentation demonstrates the ability to take a project from inception to completion, formulate and test hypotheses, and communicate knowledge from research activities. Manuscripts published in peer-reviewed journals are the ultimate proof of research excellence, as this generally involves an objective review process with experts in the field. International and national conferences are also assets, including when you were the presenter or a contributing author. Written reports, such as undergraduate honors reports, and theses, both at the bachelor's or master's level, are other structured works that are produced based on results verifying hypotheses. Personal evaluations and narrative comments provided for these entries are important to be mentioned, when applicable.

During their undergraduate or graduate degrees, applicants may have had the opportunity to compete for funding. These funding opportunities might have been summer undergraduate or graduate scholarships, at the institutional, state, provincial, or federal levels. Being awarded research funding demonstrates the ability to write and propose compelling research projects, further adding to a competitive dossier as a graduate research program applicant. Even if MD-PhD students typically receive a stipend from the university, having the potential to receive additional scholarships is important. Previously awarded research scholarships demonstrate the potential to be productive, to establish feasible research goals, and to communicate research projects and impact effectively. If possible, one must aim to obtain the most competitive scholarships, across different funding levels. In the CV, different details about the scholarships can be included, such as the funding institution, amount, duration, and the competition involved.

Finally, it is normally possible to include a section on hobbies and passions in the CV. Examples may include sports, arts, or entrepreneurial endeavors. This is a unique section that allows you to demonstrate how you maintain a balanced lifestyle and other passions outside of academic training and work. It shows that in addition to having the capacity to provide good care to patients, you can maintain a healthy work-life balance and take care of yourself throughout your academic training and future career.

Preparing the personal narrative

If you feel you still have trouble with the broader formulation of a personal narrative or the technical components of writing, refer to the section on writing application essays in Chapter 6. This section is about the content you should fit into your narrative. The application to the PhD component may include additional documents, namely a personal narrative, a list of publications, and letters of reference (typically ranging from two to three letters, depending on the institution). The personal narrative consists of a letter of intent in which you convey to the selection committee your interest in applying to the joint program, and explain why you are interested in the joint program and why you would be an excellent candidate. The narrative should include research experiences (internships, research projects, or formal degrees), as well as any inclination to conduct scientific research during medical school and in your future career as a physician-scientist. Oral and poster presentations may also be included with research publications. Moreover, you may include your area of interest for future PhD studies in this narrative as well.

The different possibilities of graduate programs and supervisors at the host institution should be examined in advance. Naming specific research programs and potential supervisors can contribute positively to the narrative. It demonstrates that you have a specific and realistic plan in mind, together with feasible goals. Even if research plans do change along the way, the fact that you are able to establish long-term goals with your future MD-PhD studies early on demonstrates the ability to do the same with subsequent research interests and projects. For example, in my case, I was pursuing master's studies in human genetics at the time. During the PhD interview, I explained how I planned on using my master's research work to develop my PhD research project. My career plans have changed; in fact, I have changed research fields. Nonetheless, being able to plan ahead for my PhD with so many specific details had shown that I knew how to create opportunities for myself, tailor my research degree to my career and life goals, and accomplish these in a timely fashion. In terms of more distant long-term goals, you may mention where you see yourself in 10 or 20 years as a physician-scientist.

Finally, it is crucial to justify choosing to pursue a joint MD-PhD program instead of solely one or the other, or both in a consecutive manner. Some medical school applicants have a PhD degree, while other medical graduates will obtain a PhD later on in their career, during a fellowship, for example. Combining a medical degree with a PhD degree is one of many ways to obtain both degrees. It is often financially compensated and is seen as very prestigious, since only a select few are chosen to pursue a joint MD-PhD program. Overall, this personal narrative is your chance to convey how motivated, determined, and passionate you are about doing both clinical and research training programs.

List of publications

The list of publications demonstrates your research track record. While not necessary, admissions committees look favorably upon early career publications in peer-reviewed journals. In the list of publications, you can highlight your position in the author list so that reviewers can easily see what the contribution is. Published conference proceedings may also count towards publications if you have not published any other manuscripts at the time of application. Inquiring directly with the university admissions committee is best to clarify any questions regarding what may be considered published work.

Asking for letters of reference

Reference letters from individuals who have acted as mentors for research activities may be used by the selection committee for both the medical and PhD applications, depending on the application requirements of the host university. It is advantageous to choose referees who have supervised you in a research project in the past and who can attest to your abilities both as a future physician and future scientist. The referees will have the opportunity to highlight, in addition to the personal narrative, any accomplishments both in and outside the laboratory, including extracurricular activities conducted with them.

Previous supervisors who know you well and who had a positive work experience with you can act as good referees. They should be able to attest to your strengths and weaknesses, accomplishments within their laboratories, factors that distinguish you from other members of the laboratory or from other colleagues, and reasons that make you an excellent candidate for an MD-PhD program. If several options of referees are possible, you may select them based on the ultimate goal of showing diversity in terms of universities, affiliations, or research fields in your application. Choosing well-known research investigators from the university itself or world-renowned experts in a specific field should also be prioritized over other research investigators. Nonetheless, it is worth mentioning that a world-renowned investigator may provide a weak reference, while a lesser-known investigator may provide you with a stellar reference.

Asking referees for letters should be done several weeks in advance, ideally four to eight weeks. It is also a good idea to remind the referee throughout this period of the reference letter and the deadline. When asking for a reference letter by email, the criteria of evaluation, the goal, and the due date of the letter should be specified in the email. Specific documentation may be sent with the request email in order to aid the referee writing the letter, including meaningful and substantial information. For example, I provided my referee with my CV, my transcript, and a summary of my research activities and contributions. I also included the list of criteria that is required for the letter based the university's rules. If the request for a reference letter is done in person, it is a good idea to follow up by email afterward. The submission deadline for the referee should be clearly indicated in the email or can be chosen to be a few days before the real deadline. This will be useful if delays occur. Friendly reminders can be sent on days closer to the submission date. As application deadlines are not flexible, referees must submit their letters on time, and it is your responsibility to ensure that the entire application package is received on time and by the set deadline.

As mentioned above, it is important to provide referees with a CV and summary of personal accomplishments when asking for reference letters. These documents may be provided in the first email that is requesting the letter or in follow-up emails when they have confirmed their support. The list of personal accomplishments that can be provided in addition to the

CV may be of particular use to them, especially if they had limited encounters with you. Some referees might ask you to draft a reference letter in advance of time for them. Therefore, it is important that you plan on having sufficient time to prepare your own supporting documents in addition to the reference letters. As previously described, you can distribute the qualities and skills from the preestablished list across your CV and personal narrative, and also across the reference letters, to ensure having a complete representation of your most valuable aptitudes throughout all the different documents submitted for the application.

THE INTERVIEW PROCESS

The interview can take the form of formal interviews with different faculty members, scenarios with actors, or solving logical reasoning problems. The standardized Multiple Mini Interview (MMI) is one type of interviews that was pioneered at McMaster in 2002 and has been adopted afterward at other schools across Canada, the United States, and internationally. Moreover, a separate interview may be conducted with the applicants for the PhD portion of the MD-PhD application.

Medical school Multiple Mini Interviews

MMIs may be one of the main components of medical school interviews. That was my experience applying to McGill University in 2017. MMIs are composed of approximately 10 different stations arranged in a circuit. They can take different forms, such as discussions with an evaluator, scenarios with actors plus hidden evaluators, or task-oriented scenarios with or without an evaluator present. They involve reallife situations that are not linked to health care or to the medical field. Medical knowledge is not expected in those scenarios, but critical thinking, empathy, listening skills, and good judgment, among others, very much are. The scenarios test human abilities and skills. It can be informative to read on those roles before preparing for the MMIs to get a sense of what is expected and evaluated for the MMIs. In addition, there are some rest stations. These are the same length as the evaluated scenarios and allow for breaks. It should be stressed that these are called rest stations for a reason. They should not be used as a time to ruminate over your own performance in the preceding MMI stations. Instead, take advantage of this time to relax and enjoy the experience.

You must be very careful when assessing how the university of choice evaluates and ranks applicants. For example, in my case at McGill University, the score from the interview (MMI) performance was combined with a McGill-calculated GPA assigned for basic science courses undertaken during my first year of studies after high school. In this particular case, the interview performance weighed more than the basic science courses. However, if the basic science courses did not have a good GPA related to them, it could have negatively affected my total post-interview score. If some basic science courses have a particularly low GPA performance, you might consider repeating those courses during summer semesters to improve the total post-interview score at upcoming application cycles.

There are a multitude of ways to prepare for the interviews. For example, you may use your already submitted CV and assign skills, lessons, and successes for each of the activities or experiences stated on the CV. This provides you with a bank of in-depth answers to aid during the interview process. It offers a way to reflect back on personal experiences and how these led to the development of specific abilities. By having in your mind the array of experiences and lessons learned throughout your life, you may have the capacity to relate more easily to other people's personal experiences as well. This is useful for both the medical school interview experience and for life in general.

Other methods of preparation include doing mock circuit interviews with friends and family. The format, length, and content can be mimicked based on how the university interviews are described. This allows you to practice the concept and sequence of interviewing at different consecutive interview stations, for example, and to understand the fast pace that is intrinsic to the process when this format is used.

There are also different strategies that can be used toward succeeding at the MMIs. Talking to upper year students that were successful in MMIs can be helpful to get input on how to prepare and what to focus on, within limits. Applicants who go through the interviews may sign a nondisclosure agreement, preventing them from sharing information that is not on the university website, such as the content of the interviews or the questions that were asked. Information sessions about the interview process, hosted by the schools of interest or by other universities or colleges assisting their own students in the process, are very helpful to understand what the admissions committee typically looks for in potential applications. In specific cases, there are also information sessions held for the unsuccessful applicants of previous application cycles.

With regard to online resources, some online programs advertise to provide help, guidance, or even coaching to perform well on the MMIs. Other programs provide visual aids, videos, and examples of typical questions and answers that can be accessed by a user, either as a trial or upon payment of a certain fee. This can be helpful to get a structured preview of interview or MMI answers. If you don't obtain an offer of admission following the interviews or MMIs, some universities will provide, upon request, the interview or MMI score of applications. Use it to improve and rank higher when reapplying during the subsequent years. Above all, remember to be professional, ethical, empathetic, and natural throughout the interviews.

PhD interview

For the PhD portion of the interview, you may be asked to present yourself in an oral presentation lasting a few minutes. You start with an introduction: who you are, your hometown, family, education background, and hobbies. The research profile is key and will consist of completed research projects, awarded scholarships, publications, and presentations. Presenting a plan for future MD-PhD studies is useful, as previously explained, to demonstrate to the faculty that precise research goals and activities have been thought about carefully and can be planned for once admitted in the program. As mentioned previously, showing your ability to conduct research projects from start to finish is crucial to convince the selection committee that the applicant will exhibit research excellence once admitted to the MD-PhD program.

Members of the committee may also take the opportunity to ask questions regarding previous extracurricular accomplishments, previous research projects, or future PhD studies. Answers about those topics should be anticipated and prepared for in advance. Showing how you will accomplish your long-term goals is essential for the selection committee to assess your ability to pursue productive MD-PhD studies. The future PhD project topic, the laboratory, and the researcher's name can be explicitly mentioned, if you have this information at the time of application. This will demonstrate your ability to efficiently plan research endeavors and to be productive during your PhD degree, which has a unique and limited time frame before the graduation deadline.

Show commitment to the joint program specifically, which is longer than just doing a medical or PhD degree alone. Perseverance and determination can be demonstrated using examples of previous personal experiences or describing motivation for pursuing this kind of joint program.

POSSIBLE OUTCOMES

After going through the application and interview process, there are five different possible outcomes.

1. You are accepted into the joint MD-PhD program.
2. You are accepted into the MD program only.
3. You are placed on a waiting list for the joint MD-PhD program.
4. You are placed on a waiting list for the MD program only.
5. You are not accepted to either MD-PhD or MD programs.

If option 2 occurs, you may have the opportunity to apply to the MD-PhD program as a first-year medical student, depending on the university. The priority should be to get into the MD program, as this is often the roadblock for MD-PhD applicants. If options 3, 4, or 5 arise, remind yourself that the process of applying and interviewing is an important learning experience in itself. You learn a lot about yourself, your abilities, and perseverance through the preparation of your application. It will be important for you to understand why the application was refused or waitlisted and at what stage this happened. Whether you were refused pre-interview or post-interview will determine how to better prepare for the subsequent application cycle. The priority should be to get into the MD program, as this is often the roadblock for MD-PhD applicants.

When reapplying to the subsequent cycles of applications, previous documents can be used again and importantly, be improved. Have other individuals read through the application documents, whether it be people that know you on a personal or professional basis. During the subsequent year after a refusal, it will be important to get involved in different activities that bring new assets, values, and other qualities. Widening your research endeavors, publishing results, or presenting at conferences might help prove research potential. Starting a research-based master's degree may also offer additional experiences that are beneficial when applying to a combined MD-PhD degree, both for academic productivity and eligibility reasons.

CONCLUSION

I hope you found this overview of the application process useful and enlightening. Throughout the process, remember that many people do apply multiple times to either medical or joint MD-PhD programs before being successful and obtaining an offer of admission. The years spent perfecting personal abilities and acquiring additional academic training before being accepted should not be seen as obstacles, but as unique opportunities to live enriching experiences and gain maturity and knowledge that will prepare you to become a successful physician-scientist. I personally learned a lot about myself, my qualities and flaws, and how I have transformed past life experiences into learning experiences. Preparing an application to an MD-PhD program is an accomplishment on its own because of its diverse demands, and every step taken successfully during the application process should be celebrated.

Part II

Early Days in Medical School

8

Starting Medical School and Integrating Research

Heather T. Whittaker

Heather T. Whittaker is a fourth-year MD PhD student at McGill University, where she is researching the effects of noninvasive brain stimulation on memory processes as a therapeutic approach for people with neurocognitive decline. She previously studied at the University of Winnipeg (BS in biopsychology) and University College London (MS in clinical neuroscience).

INTRODUCTION

Congratulations, you've turned the page to a new chapter of your life—the beginning of your training as a physician-scientist! The corresponding chapter of this book is meant to help you orient yourself amidst all of the excitement and the uncertainty of beginning medical school and chart a course for the long journey ahead. Maybe you already have a concrete plan for the next 8 years of school before residency. For that, I admire you. Maybe you tend to take things one step at a time and, like me, are wondering how to shift your focus now that you've gained acceptance to your dream program. Whoever you are, now is a good time to pause and reflect on your accomplishments, evaluate your goals, and most importantly, celebrate.

You've worked long and hard to get to this point, to be selected amongst thousands of highly qualified applicants and earn a place in your program. This achievement cannot be understated and should not be downplayed. Relish the feeling that your future as a physician-scientist is now more tangible than ever. Becoming an MD-PhD trainee brings

---

WHAT YOU NEED TO KNOW

- Get to know your classmates and surround yourself with supportive people.
- Consider altering your study strategy and expectations for exams.
- Say yes to learning opportunities and keep an open mind about what interests you.
- Search for a career mentor who inspires you professionally and personally.
- Focus on establishing and maintaining healthy habits in your personal life.

both a well-deserved sense of security and the humbling knowledge that ever-greater challenges lie on the horizon. Life may not get any easier from here on, but it will hopefully become more rewarding as you develop your dual career and begin to apply your knowledge and skills to improve patient care. It will be critical to your well-being and success that you learn to pace yourself. In moments of uncertainty, remember how you felt reading Chapter 1 ("Is the MD-PhD Path Right for You?") of this book, and be reassured that you are in a supportive program that exists to help you flourish.

BUILDING A NETWORK

The single best piece of advice I can give to first-year medical students is to spend more time getting to know your classmates and less time comparing yourself to them. These two deceptively simple objectives will enhance both your professional and personal growth. The benefits of making strong connections with classmates extend beyond your social fulfillment; these people will be your support network in medical school and your future colleagues in clinical practice. It's unrealistic to try making friends with everyone, but you should at least make a point to know as many of your classmates as possible. If you will leave your class after second year for PhD studies, keep in mind that by the time you return to medical school, your entering cohorts will be senior students who can be valuable sources of advice on the wards and with residency programs. Additionally, you should make an effort to connect with your fellow MD-PhD students. One of the greatest advantages of being in a joint degree program is the opportunity to befriend other students at all levels of MD-PhD training, as they will have the best understanding of the hurdles that await and the most relevant tips to overcome them.

As you get to know your peers better, it can be tempting to harbor feelings of inadequacy. By virtue of making it through the fine filters of medical school admissions, the students in your class will have impressive extracurricular engagements, more varied work experience, and many more Olympic medals than you. At all costs, resist succumbing to imposter syndrome, and remember that you've been given the opportunity to learn with and from this group of people. Looking around at your classmates, you will realize that you all genuinely want each other to be the best physicians possible. To this aim, you are all going to do what you can to help each other out; this is especially true if your school has a pass-fail grading scheme, which can reduce competition between students and encourage collaboration. A healthy dose of humility will serve you well, but you must not forget your own exceptional capabilities.

STARTING MEDICAL SCHOOL

The truth is that in medical school, as in your previous education, there is no secret formula for succeeding academically. You will have to design a strategy that works for you. I will do my best to provide you with a framework to do this, but let me first tell you a bit about my own experience. I came to medical school after a graduate degree and a year of full-time employment, so I can speak to the challenge of returning to classes after some time off. I received my notice of admission in the summer of 2017, after a few harrowing months on the waiting list. I was thrilled to get to move to Montreal, a vibrant city that also happened to be home to a university with a great medical program and a storied neurological institute. My first month in the city was a whirlwind of exploring its many summer festivals and attractions, settling into a new apartment, and starting medical school.

As I eased myself back into student life, my energy was not entirely devoted to my studies, but I figured that my enthusiasm for learning would return soon enough. This was an attitude that persisted throughout my first year. I had an overwhelming sense of being in over my head with schoolwork, a declining motivation to study, and an apprehension that I would forget most of what I learned during the intervening PhD years. I told myself that because I had put in so much effort to maintain a perfect GPA during undergrad, it was good for me to slow down now that I had gotten into a program where the grades didn't matter. After all, the student who finishes last in medical school is still a qualified doctor at the end of the day, right? In retrospect, I think I was afflicted with was a form of burnout—I stopped listening to lectures and came very close to failing exams.

This story is not meant to be a cautionary tale about the dangers of falling behind in medical school. Rather, I think it illustrates that you needn't become discouraged if you don't excel right out of the gate. That is a theme I will emphasize in this chapter: Becoming a physician takes time, so be patient and trust the process. In an address to medical students, Sir William Osler wrote that The hardest conviction to get into the mind of a beginner is that the education upon which he is engaged is not a college course, not a medical course, but a life course, for which the work of a few years under teachers is but a preparation. My professors likened learning in pre-clerkship to drinking from a firehose. You simply cannot absorb all of the material you will be given to study, and you must not be put off by this. Although you may not understand every lecture slide at the start, you'll be thinking like a physician before you know it with repeated exposure to patterns of disease presentation and clinical problem solving. Laying down the foundations of medicine is important in the first and second year—even in a combined MD-PhD program—but the real high-yield learning happens on the wards, when you see things in their clinical context, over and over and over.

Preclinical studies

Since you've made it into medical school, you've likely optimized a personal study strategy. That said, the sort of studying you will do during your preclinical years differs considerably from the studying you did during your undergraduate degree. There are a few key reasons why you may want to try alternate methods.

First, there are probably going to be exams every few weeks throughout the year, rather than a week of testing at the end of each semester. With this structure, it can be tempting to selectively study the most testable material, but you mustn't lose sight of the larger picture. Your aim should not be to simply score highly on exams and promptly forget the material thereafter. This is knowledge that you will use in the care of patients, directly or indirectly, and it is your job to eventually become competent with all of the learning objectives. Rather than strategically omitting certain subjects and focusing on exam-relevant hints from lecturers, try to spend your study time reading into areas where your understanding is weak.

In addition, most schools design their course modules to fit together and build upon one another in a cohesive manner. This simplifies your learning process and is also a requirement for accreditation. I personally found my preclinical curriculum, which focused on one body system at a time, easier to manage than my undergraduate course load, made up of unrelated courses on a range of subjects from chemistry to history. I appreciated that study sessions are much more streamlined in medical school.

You might also want to consider study methods that are better suited to the large volume of material given for medical school exams. Perhaps taking extremely detailed notes and writing out sections of your textbook worked for you in the past, but your time may be better spent reading and rereading information pertinent to exams. I personally reduced my in-class note-taking to only a few points that piqued my interest in class and tried to become less dependent on studying notes that I had synthesized myself. This is mainly because I envisaged myself in clerkship and residency with very little time for studying, and so I thought it would be useful to become accustomed to effectively learning via reading online and print resources. There are likely already some excellent student-generated study guides tailored to your medical school's curriculum, with handy summaries and comparison charts for rapid exam preparation.

Lastly, if you want to practice medicine in the United States, you'll want to consider preparing for the United States Medical Licensing Exam (USMLE) Step 1. More information about this standardized exam and relevant considerations for MD-PhD students can be found in Chapter 21. Briefly, most students aim to write it immediately after the preclinical phase of medical school while their basic science knowledge is strong, and before diving into more clinically oriented learning in clerkship. You may choose to incorporate USMLE Step 1 learning materials into your study strategy from the start of your first year, so that you become familiar with the popular reference books and have a complete set of your own notes for reference when it comes to dedicated study time.

The bottom line is, don't be afraid to change your study habits throughout the year as you figure out how best to organize each block of information. If you study best with other people, establish a small study group, but be prepared to switch it up if you have different approaches, such as quizzing, flashcards, or note reading. I found study groups to be efficient and improve my ability to take in information verbally, which is an important skill for future learning on the wards.

I should also mention that now is a good time to abandon the expectation to be at the top of your class. It can be hard for some students who are accustomed to A+ scores to accept an average grade, which indicates that you have in fact learned enough to be well prepared for clerkship. Indeed, there will be exam questions that you are not expected to be able to answer as a first-year medical student and require reading around your lecture notes, in order to keep the class average around 70%. Try your best, but don't be surprised if you don't manage to score the sort of grades that you did in undergraduate biology courses—it's not because you are any less smart, it's just the program adapting to a classroom full of students as smart as you.

Clinical exposure

As an MD-PhD student, you might feel prematurely pressured to align your current research interests or doctoral thesis with the branch of medicine that you imagine yourself practicing in. You might think you have a solid idea of what specialty, or even subspecialty, will be the best fit for you and your research expertise. Ultimately, mapping out your entire career at the outset of medical training is neither necessary for your success nor beneficial for your stress levels. Rest assured that you will never become trapped into a certain clinical practice just because you have a research background there. Graduates of MD-PhD programs have been known to reorient their research focus during clerkship or residency, after falling in love with a specialty outside of their previous academic experience. That doesn't make their PhD any less valuable. The various soft skills gained while completing a PhD, such as those discussed in Chapter 12 ("Maximizing Research Productivity"), are very transferable and continue to serve these physician-scientists in many ways.

The very best way to get a feel for what your future career could be like is, of course, to try it. Your school's curriculum should present you with a taste of most medical specialties, through pre-clerkship modules and clerkship rotations; there may even be patient encounters built in to your first-year courses. In addition, you can independently arrange to shadow individual physicians, which can be helpful for some students (although not necessary to succeed in medical school or as a future physician). If you feel as though you've got more than enough on your plate at the outset of medical school, don't worry about shadowing; you will spend enough time in the background of busy clinics and operating rooms as a more senior student. You will have plenty of opportunities to impress staff when you are equipped with more training and knowledge.

If you do choose to shadow during the first years of medical school, you might consider approaching physicians who have delivered a lecture to your class, either in person following the lecture, or by email shortly thereafter. Starting a conversation about what you found interesting or enjoyable about their lecture is a nice way to break the ice and will also help you identify potentially engaging specialties. Given the number of different career options within medicine, it is often a process of ruling specialties out, rather than finding "the one." There is a terrible misconception that you must begin grooming yourself from the first year of medical school in order to be a competitive applicant to residency programs. Few students are able to determine their clinical calling so early on in training. Other students may prefer to remain pluripotent until they enter clerkship and give a fair chance to a number of different departments. You are an MD-PhD student, so you have the additional opportunity to explore your options during graduate studies and perhaps sharpen your competitive edge, as detailed in Chapter 14 ("Maintaining Clinical knowledge, Skills, and Understanding During the PhD Training Years").

INTEGRATING RESEARCH

How you incorporate research during the first phase of your program will depend on whether you are continuing previous projects or starting a new project with a new lab. Some students have the option to stay in the lab where they conducted honors or master's degree work and must decide to either build directly upon that work or step into a new research arena for their doctorate. Several important aspects of this decision are considered in Chapter 10 "Selecting a Research Group and Mentor(s)", which also provides advice on contacting supervisors and sorting out a reasonable PhD project. Setting these matters aside for now, I will focus on the ways in which you can integrate research into your first and second years of medical school.

I joined the MD-PhD program at an institution where I had not previously studied, so at least one thing was certain: I needed to find a new research group. In addition to searching for a doctoral supervisor and potential projects, I was also finishing up papers from both my undergraduate and master's projects. Finding time and energy to write was surprisingly difficult after a long day of class. My undergraduate paper was especially demanding—it had received several rejections from a variety of journals, and I was facing the onerous task of reanalyzing data that I had collected years prior using methods that I was no longer familiar with. In order to finally get a publication from that project, I ended up forming an international collaboration between a physics lab and a molecular biology lab and transporting dozens of mouse brains across the Atlantic Ocean. Dedicating time to work on this project was challenging but very possible with some readjustment of my study schedule.

This was no doubt a rewarding experience, and also a taste of the time-management skills required to juggle dual commitments to research and medicine. I decided not to involve myself in any new projects with prospective PhD labs until I had wrapped up work on my previous research. However, the preclinical years of your program can be a golden opportunity to get a head start on your doctoral lab work. Chapter 15 ("Completing Your Project") provides an excellent account of the benefits of starting your PhD work early. At the very least, you should plan to test out the climate in a wide variety of labs during the first year of your program. Once you narrow in on a handful of research groups that you think might be a good fit, you might even devise a series of makeshift rotations through these groups.

FREE TIME

Ask yourself: "What activities make me feel the most like myself?" Keep doing those things, even if it means you don't have as much time to study as you think you need. It is of the utmost importance to establish healthy habits in your first year that will contribute to making you feel balanced and whole. Artistic pursuits can easily be sidelined during busy times, but you might come upon avenues for artistic expression in medical school itself—perhaps you can write poetry for a medical journal, produce a promotional video for your program, or play music at student-run charity events. If it is truly too much to keep up with your hobbies alongside studying and research, try out some ways to integrate the activities you love into the nonacademic but productive hours of your day. For example, listening to audiobooks while cooking, cleaning, or exercising can go a long way toward keeping you grounded.

You will also have the chance to join a huge array of student interest groups, including groups that are focused on a specific medical specialty and general interest clubs. You could apply for an executive position in a specialty-focused group or go to a variety of different events hosted by different clubs to get widest possible exposure to both specialties and people in your class. However you choose to spend your time, getting involved in student groups is almost always a guaranteed way to enrich your medical school experience.

CONCLUSION

For MD-PhD students, the first 2 years of medical school can be a chance to prepare for the upcoming marathon of research and clinical training. Your experience will depend on how you divide your time between studying course material, advancing research projects, and personal interests. What will invariably make your experience more enjoyable and memorable is making connections with the people you share it with.

9

Strategizing Your Research Rotations for Success

Justin Lowenthal · Ethan Cottrill

Justin Lowenthal *is a seventh-year MD-PhD student at Johns Hopkins University. His PhD research is in biomedical engineering, co-mentored between two advisors and two different labs, and centers on using stem cells, genetics, developmental biology, and tissue engineering techniques to model cardiac development and genetic heart disease. Prior to medical school, Justin completed a bachelor of science in biomedical engineering from Yale University and a certificate in bioethics at the National Institutes of Health.*

Ethan Cottrill *is a fifth-year MD-PhD student at Johns Hopkins University. His PhD research is in biomedical engineering and centers on developing new bone graft substitute materials. Prior to medical school, Ethan completed a bachelor of science in chemistry from Ohio University and a master of science in education from Johns Hopkins University.*

INTRODUCTION

Research rotations, where early graduate students get an abbreviated but immersive experience in a lab that is under their consideration for PhD thesis work, are an exciting part of MD-PhD training. Because in many cases everything is suddenly new again—the

WHAT YOU NEED TO KNOW

- Before and during a rotation, prioritize collecting the data you need to determine if it is the right home for you and your PhD training over productivity.
- Conversations with program directors and upper-year students, as well as thorough searching of available online and local resources, can help you identify potential mentors and labs in which to rotate.
- Make sure to consider both objective measures of a lab's success and subjective experiences in that lab—both your own during the rotation, and the experiences of those who are currently in the lab and those who may have chosen to go elsewhere.
- Have many conversations and ask many questions during your rotation, inside and outside the lab, to get the most out of the experience.
- Ending a lab rotation can be awkward, but it is important to be transparent, respectful, and clear, expressing gratitude for the experience and your plan moving forward regardless of your decision.

environment, the people, the research—research rotations often create a "honeymoon" period for the budding scientist, marked with significant growth, fulfillment, and learning. These typically 6- to 10-week experiences allow early graduate students to appreciate and absorb the science and culture of discovery and mentorship in a lab without the responsibility of committing to the lab or dedicating oneself to a project. With that said, rotation students can make significant contributions to the lab, though the weeks- to months-long time frame obviously poses some constraints on what can be achieved, and productivity should not be the primary goal.

The next chapter in this book focuses on picking your advisor and lab following your research rotations. Here, we break down four primary subtopics: 1) the why, when, who, where, and how of research rotations; 2) maximizing value during the rotation; 3) ending a research rotation; and 4) the non-critical elements of the rotation.

THE WHY, WHEN, WHO, WHERE, AND HOW OF RESEARCH ROTATIONS

The why: Exploring your options

Would you purchase a car without first going for a test drive? Marry someone without dating for at least a bit of time? Most of us know that making such momentous decisions without a trial period would be risky. In a similar vein, the research rotation allows students to experience a lab before making a commitment. "Is this lab—the mentor, the size, the subject matter, the culture—the right fit for me? Could I see myself spending the next 4-5 years of my life here?"

Many MD-PhD students enter their programs with some degree of undergraduate and/or postbaccalaureate research experience. Despite this, research backgrounds for many students are relatively narrow in scope; our prior research work, while sufficient for motivating us to apply and making us competitive for MD-PhD programs, may not be exactly what we see ourselves wanting to do for our graduate work and/or our long-term careers. Interests change and expand, particularly for MD-PhD students as they get exposed to a deluge of new information in medical school. Furthermore, prior research experiences as undergraduates, technicians, or research assistants do not often carry with them the weight of responsibility that comes with designing and executing independent work, managing multiple projects, and ultimate ownership of a thesis that represents publishable and thematically coherent contributions to a body of work. Thus, the research rotations allow students the time to explore a wide range of research areas.

With that said, multiple factors ultimately contribute toward what lab to choose—and it should not just be limited to the type of research carried out in that lab. See Chapter 10 ("Selecting a Research Group and Mentor(s)") for more advice on making that decision.

The when: Getting to know a lab

In terms of the timing during the MD-PhD training trajectory, there is often great flexibility in setting up research rotations. In some cases, MD-PhD students are required or elect to rotate in a potential research lab during the summer before starting coursework in the fall. In other cases, students perform their first official research rotation during the summer following a year of medical school. In our experience, it is also possible to informally rotate in a lab during the academic terms of the first 2 years of medical school. Obviously, in this case, the productivity expectations are generally low because it is understood that you are mostly focused on learning the foundations of medicine. Attending lab meetings during the medical school years and reading the literature from labs you think you may be interested in are excellent ways to become involved in a lab early on. When you perform your research rotations is also ultimately dependent on how you decide to structure your training. For example, completing 2 years of medical school and then starting the PhD is most typical, but other orders of PhD and MD training are possible and sometimes pursued, depending on what is permitted by your MD-PhD program.

Either way, most research rotations generally occur during the first year of PhD training. In most cases, the length of the rotation is mutually agreed upon with the principal investigator (PI) of the lab before, or near the start of, the rotation, often with some guidance from the school registrar or PhD program administration. We recommend spending a minimum of eight weeks rotating in a lab, which we believe is generally enough time to adequately get to know the dynamics of the lab and decide whether you can see yourself in that lab for 3 or more years. Because most PhD programs expect students to join a lab by the end of their first year in the PhD program—in some cases, because of funding or training grant requirements—it is generally advisable to be diligent regarding the timing of your research rotations. If you are really having fun and enjoying your time in the lab, it may be best to stay longer (or even commit to the lab early, if allowed by your PhD program). If you decide early on during the rotation that the lab is definitely not the right lab for you, then there is no real use in continuing in the lab, and it may be best to talk with the PI about an early exit from your rotation.

The who and where: Discovering your interests and needs

How do you identify mentors for considerations and labs for possible rotations? This varies a bit by your institution (and any other academic, medical, or nonprofit institutions linked to it) and your research interests, but there are some important general principles. Having a broad conversation with your MD-PhD program director as well as the PhD program director(s) of the program(s) you are considering is incredibly useful. You can discuss your research interests, your priorities in a mentor, what you know about yourself and how you work, and what things are still not certain for you. The directors can share their knowledge of labs, discuss the experiences of students training in labs of potential interest, identify labs, mentors, or departments that you may not have identified yourself, and share their insight about the status of a lab (e.g., funding, whether it might be moving, what collaborations they have). They might even identify connections between your research interests and provide insights that redirect your thinking regarding research areas.

Similar conversations can and should be had with upper-level students in the program who are in or have completed their PhD training, particularly those who have worked or are working in labs you might consider. Some programs will have formal mechanisms for doing this—for example, a panel of graduate students, meet-and-greet programs, research retreats, lists of students and their mentors for contact—but word-of-mouth can be a powerful tool (as can the advice of experienced administrators in your program).

Beyond these conversations, it is often helpful to take a broad approach to searching for potential labs, as websites and other tools for searching all of the various labs and faculty in an institution or department can vary widely in quality, user-friendliness, and comprehensiveness. Starting your search from the websites of graduate programs that interest you to find their affiliated faculty is important, but make sure to look at websites of the broader departments, special research institutes, other affiliated institutions, or collaborative centers. Clinical department websites (through their research pages) can be great resources as well. Even the news section of your institutions can be searched by subject matter/scientific topic to see which labs have recently published or made news around a topic.

The Internet can be a huge resource here. Searching topics of interest with the name of your institution using Google, Google Scholar, and PubMed can be helpful (make sure to use different phrases, combinations of words, and append the names of institutions that are affiliated with your program). Websites such as Pure (Elsevier) and ScienceDirect often have the ability to search by institution, to find any and all scientists who have published on that topic who were or are affiliated with an institution, often with metrics on productivity over time. Scientific journals/publications of relevance to your field as well as general-interest scientific journals can often be searched by institution as well. Social media—Twitter, in particular— can often be mined (using hashtags and networks to known scientists) for ideas, particularly in recent years where scientists have been more engaged in publicizing their work through these channels. Finally, for American institutions, NIH RePORTER will often list labs that are funded for particular topics via federal funding, and Grantome will often have a similar resource and include other sources of funding. Statewide or nonprofit associations that provide funding will have lists of their grantees that can be searched as well.

This may all sound very overwhelming—it is completely okay to keep your search minimal and your list short, or to even know going in where you want to rotate and forego searching entirely. Often, students embarking on finding rotation labs will keep a spreadsheet of their own with information on labs that interest them, the mentors, the research areas in those labs, and notes on any "intangibles" gleaned from conversations with other students, program directors, or even meetings with the faculty members themselves. When it comes time to narrow down and make a choice, try to limit the number of meetings you set up with labs and faculty of interest, have a set of questions that you want to know the answers to before rotating, and record your impressions immediately afterward. Otherwise, too many meetings and too few notes can cause these meetings to run together and your impressions to be forgotten among the other things you are doing in medical school. It is good practice to send a prompt thank-you message after a meeting and be transparent about your intentions—whether to rotate in the lab (and along what timeline) and/or whether you plan to keep searching before you decide.

It is important to keep in mind whether having a mentor or mentors who are themselves physician-scientists (with an MD or MD-PhD vs. PhD training) is important to you, as some will value having a mentor whom they can emulate and learn balancing clinical and research obligations from directly. Often a physician-scientist will be familiar with the rigors and timelines of your training in a way that a PhD (particularly if inexperienced) will not. However, PhDs can be and often are phenomenal mentors and do important, clinically relevant work; sometimes it requires rotating and evaluating the relationship itself rather than prematurely limiting your possible mentors based on this factor alone. Similarly, seniority is often a consideration for students—faculty who are more senior may have more experience in mentorship and more established track records in a field, both for publication and for placing trainees. That said, junior faculty can sometimes be more engaged in your work, as it may be critical for their funding and tenure promotion. These generalizations do not always hold, and there are pros and cons to working in labs large and small, with senior versus junior faculty.

Remember to keep your eyes, ears, and mind open! Your first 2 years of medical school are a deluge of new information, and you may find a particular topic or clinical application (or lecturer) engaging and interesting in ways you did not foresee. Use your medical school courses and lectures as a resource to identify your own interests as well as potential labs and mentors. Keeping your eyes open to bulletin boards, email lists, and online calendars for lectures happening around campus can allow you to see a researcher (or one of their trainees) give a presentation on what their lab is doing; these are invaluable for getting a personal sense of whether the topic is enthralling and the mentor "clicks" for you. Additionally, embrace change! Your interests may shift during the first 2 years of medical school, both within a scientific discipline and between disciplines (even away from basic science toward more clinical/public health or vice versa). Use your rotations to experience a variety of environments, of course, but also a variety of topic areas and scientific techniques to see what feels engaging to you. It is a journey.

The next chapter, which addresses the final choice of lab and mentor and the considerations that play into it, is also worth looking at. You should be thinking ahead; your primary goal in your research rotations is, after all, to consider a potential future in these labs.

The how: Approaching, shadowing, and acclimating

In most cases, setting up a research rotation is straightforward: you contact the lab in some way (generally by sending an email to the PI), meet with the PI, and agree upon the logistics of the rotation. When meeting with the PI, it is common to talk about lab projects, including which you find most interesting and where you would like to become involved. From our experience, it's also common for rotation students to spend the first couple of weeks in the lab "shadowing" different graduate students, postdoctoral fellows, and/or other lab personnel to learn more about the different ongoing projects.

Following this initial shadowing period, it is expected that students will pick an area of interest for focus during the rotation and work closely with the graduate student leading that research area. In some cases, rotation students may also want to lead their own small projects during the research rotation. These students should keep in mind the time constraints of a research rotation as well as the lab's overall interest in expanding into new areas (especially considering the risk that the rotation student may not commit to the lab). Otherwise, rotation students generally work in the lab on a schedule similar to any other first- or second-year graduate student who has already committed to the lab (keeping in mind that these students—whether committed or also rotating—may be concurrently taking classes and are mostly on a learning curve themselves). In the following section, we discuss ways to maximize value during the research rotation.

MAXIMIZING VALUE DURING THE ROTATION

As mentioned, and as discussed further in Chapter 10, there is much to consider when embarking upon a rotation—much data to gather, only some of which is at the lab bench.

Objective measures of a lab's success are critical, and sometimes the best way to get access to this information is by rotating in the lab itself. Time to graduation, funding availability and sources (both public and private, large and small, and institutional and individ fellowships), track record of graduates, and publication history are all important and helpful to ascertain. Less obvious but arguably equally important questions to ask include: What types of projects is the lab undertaking, and how many are collaborative with other labs? Are there many co-senior-authored and/or co-first-authored publications? How are lab meetings structured, and do they seem engaging and productive for the lab? Are trainees afforded opportunities to travel and present their work, to make connections with important members of the scientific and institutional communities, and to take time off to recharge and for personal growth?

To this end, objective metrics start to blur into the subjective. This is where spending as much time interacting with the mentor(s) in the lab—both directly in regular meetings, and indirectly by observing their interactions with other trainees, colleagues, and staff—is of utmost priority during a rotation. Seek to set up a regular meeting with the PI of the lab in which you are rotating, both to go over any scientific progress and also to talk more generally about research, their view of the science being pursued, their philosophy on running their lab and on mentoring trainees, questions that you've had about the science and the field more generally, and more.

Join in on lab meetings and any smaller group meetings within the lab relevant to your interests. Watch how the PI and other senior members of the lab—research faculty, staff scientists, postdoctoral fellows, and senior staff—run the lab and use positive or negative feedback with the more junior trainees. Ask about collaborative projects and relationships with other labs—particularly if you are interested in a jointly advised, co-mentored PhD—to see if there are ways to become involved in that work.

Use every opportunity to have conversations, formal and informal, with others in the lab at all levels of their training. The true value of a rotation is the opportunity to drill down and get the lived experiences of those who are immersed in it daily. Ask questions, both substantive and seemingly trivial. The questions might include these examples: "Do you have the flexibility to work at the hours you choose? Do you feel that your mentor is actively promoting your individual professional development and is sensitive to your personal well-being, or are they focused purely on advancing the science? Are you able to get the resources, materials, and information you need? What resources and facilities on campus does the lab make use of? Is the lab social? Do lab members spend time with one another outside of the lab and lab activities? What do you like best and dislike most about the PI?"

Make sure to have as many conversations with members of the lab outside of the setting of the lab (and lab-related activities) as possible. Often lab members will feel external or even internal pressure to be in "recruitment mode" when in the laboratory setting, particularly if they are motivated to recruit a new, energetic, enthusiastic, and collegial lab member to work with them on their project(s). Conversations outside of the lab—for example, over coffee, at meals off-site, at conferences, or at informal social activities—to probe for the true feelings of the lab member about their project, the strengths and weaknesses of their mentor(s), what they would change about how the lab is run or the science is done—can be the most revealing part of a lab rotation. If possible, it is even worthwhile to ask to speak to graduates/alumni of the lab about their perspectives on the lab and the mentor, as well as any trainees who have rotated in and elected not to join or decided to leave the lab, to determine whether the lab and the mentor are indeed a good fit and to elicit any red flags.

Finally and more broadly, a research rotation is a graduate student's first opportunity to gain true insight into the broader institutional culture: the attitude around rotations, whether labs or departments tend to be collegial or closed off and "siloed," and whether there is a larger community of scientists dedicated to free exchange at the institution in the scientific field of interest. Pay close attention to your instincts and feelings about the lab, the department, the research community, and the PI. Ask yourself: If you were running this lab, what would you do differently? Is this lab at the right place on the spectrum of engaged and hands-on, to hands-off and fostering independence? Do certain personalities and perspectives dominate lab discussions, or is there a true openness to diverse ideas and a tolerance for objection, constructive critique, and well-reasoned but unintentional error? Are the trainees diverse in background, demographics, and expertise, and if not, is there a reason why?

Rotations are an opportunity to ask all your questions—small and large, substantive and trivial, professional and personal, conceptual and technical—without consequence. Use it to its fullest.

ENDING A RESEARCH ROTATION

Ending a research rotation can be tough—so much so that we elected to write about this as its own subtopic. From the PI's point of view, there are few things more disheartening in research than openly welcoming a promising rotation student into the lab; providing the student with time, money, and other resources; and giving the student a first-hand look at the lab's most important ideas and methods—all for the rotation student to decline the lab and take their newfound knowledge and skills elsewhere. It is for this reason that some labs won't accept rotation students unless they commit to the lab even before starting their rotation/PhD work. For these reasons, deciding to end the research rotation should be a carefully calculated decision—and one filled with expressed appreciation to the PI for the opportunity.

Regardless of the reason for deciding to end the rotation, we strongly caution against burning any bridges with the PI or lab members, as people generally remember how you treat them—and you obviously don't want your professional reputation to be described as poor by anyone. The PI and/or their lab may be a future collaborator, thesis committee member, study section reviewer, or manuscript editor.

The best defense here is a good offense. In most cases, communicating to the PI at the start of the rotation that you want to rotate in another lab after theirs can set expectations early and decrease sensitivities toward the end of the rotation. It is generally understandable that PhD students may want to rotate in multiple labs before choosing their PhD lab. While ultimately choosing your PhD lab/mentor is the topic of the next chapter in this book, we encourage students to express gratitude to all members of a rotation lab, and be honest and empathetic regarding your decision.

CONCLUSION

Rotating students often feel pressure to contribute immediately to a new lab, to prove themselves, to combat imposter syndrome, and to make an impact. It is easy to become immersed in a scientific subject and the importance of what you are doing in a particular field of science. You may feel the pressure to focus your rotation on having a presentation, abstract, or even publication to show for it. Ultimately, however, graduate training should prepare you not just to be good at science but to be an analytical thinker, a problem solver, a program designer, a conscientious colleague, an effective communicator, and a compassionate and dedicated mentor. No matter its level of substance, your scientific contributions during eight weeks will not help to inform you of whether this lab is the right place to land (other than, perhaps, to tell you whether, deep down, you feel engaged in the work).

Focus on determining whether by joining this lab, you will be motivated by and productive in achieving the particular research goals, able to learn what you need to be successful, and find yourself in a place that is sustainable for you personally (a healthy, energizing, nurturing environment for your particular set of needs). To put it simply, you have one goal during a research rotation: introspection. Focus on your personal takeaways.

10

Selecting a Research Group and Mentor(s)

Lashanda Skerritt • Jiameng Xu

Lashanda Skerritt *is a fourth-year MD-PhD student at McGill University. Her PhD research is in family medicine and primary care, and it focuses on the reproductive health care needs and priorities of women living with HIV in Canada. Prior to medical school, Lashanda completed a bachelor of science in biochemistry from the University of Ottawa.*

Jiameng Xu *is in her sixth year of the MD-PhD program at McGill University. She completed undergraduate studies in life sciences, concentrating in neuroscience, at Queen's University in Kingston, Ontario. She has been involved in initiatives to create a space for the arts and humanities within health professional training and in spaces of health care delivery. She aims to continue writing about narrative and experience, and to dedicate herself to working with patients and their families.*

INTRODUCTION

In a discussion with a friend facing the decision of whether she should stay in her current research group or transfer to a different one, I began thinking of our research groups as a series of villages. When joining a village, for the next 3–4 years you will be tasked with learning their language, customs, values, and traditions. The neighbors of the village, both near and far, will also become your neighbors and ultimately your network. Therefore, it is important to select a village that can help you, as a student, answer the questions that you want to study. It is perhaps easier if the village is already asking questions similar to your questions, indicating a shared

---

WHAT YOU NEED TO KNOW

- Consider how you have learned and performed best in the past, and what you want to accomplish and learn as a PhD student.
- Speak to current and former students to determine how you would fit with a specific supervisor or research environment.
- Invest time preparing for your meetings with potential supervisors. Use this chapter to develop your list of questions.
- Be ready to be flexible with your thesis research project and expectations.
- Search for a supervisor that can help you achieve your broader education and career goals.

interest. You should also feel welcomed and accepted by the village; it is difficult to thrive in a hostile village. It is also vital that the country where the village is located is safe, stable, and has adequate resources; a research group can be very attractive, but if the department is facing overarching issues, such as a lack of funding, that will affect you as well.

Much like choosing a village, choosing your research lab necessarily raises some important questions: "Do I want to learn their language, and customs? Will they accept the values and traditions I have learned from my previous village and help me to develop my skills further? Would I enjoy living in this village for the next couple of years?"

The village we arrive in is not always the village we settle in. Physician-scientists may hold dual or multiple citizenships. They may also be nomadic and choose not to settle in any single village or disciplinary community at all. Perhaps there is a village in the future that one would like to get to, but it is not currently accessible, and choosing to do a PhD in a particular village that is more accessible can be a stepping stone to reaching or establishing this village in the future. Time spent in a village leaves its mark on us, and because of this, exposure to different and sometimes unanticipated villages is valuable.

Much like your decision to apply to an MD-PhD program, choosing a supervisor, research group, and project requires self-reflection. Two questions that can help to guide this reflection are: 1) What are your goals for your PhD and research career? 2) What type of supervisor and research environment will help you achieve those goals?

PREPARE FOR SELF-REFLECTION

Your interests and priorities will help to inform your answer to the first question: What do you want out of your PhD? This chapter is intended to highlight some important considerations as you decide on the village you will settle in. In an MD-PhD training program, your doctoral research is expected to make a novel and meaningful contribution to your area of interest, applying the language, methodologies, and contexts in that field. In addition to your contribution to the field, your doctoral studies also provide opportunities for your personal and career development, such as training in different methodological approaches, and developing professional skills. Your PhD should, additionally, provide opportunities for teamwork and network building, all of which will help to support your career as a physician-scientist.

When you are deciding on a supervisor and research group, there are a few points to help frame your decision-making process. The first is to decide how you will identify the supervisor(s) that best fits with your learning style. The second is to determine the type of supervisory relationship you will need to flourish during your doctoral studies. Third, you must consider how your doctoral supervisor will support you in pursuing your career goals. Your supervisor does not have to be a role model for your future career. In fact, their career might be quite different from what you envision for yourself. Regardless, your supervisor should support you in your development as a researcher and help you achieve your career goals.

IDENTIFYING POTENTIAL SUPERVISORS

There are various ways you can identify putative PhD supervisors. You may identify supervisors from the recommendations of your mentors or previous supervisors. Perhaps you've met researchers at conferences and seminars whose work interests you. Potential supervisors may also be identified through the websites of your prospective institution. Productive researchers with a good track record of publications and supervising graduate students are ideal, but it's worth noting that some PhD students go on to have impressive academic careers after being the very first graduate student supervised by an early-career researcher. There is no single formula for success, and what works for you may be very different from what works for someone else. Generally, thesis supervisors are important for several expansive reasons: 1) they provide direction on your thesis, 2) they provide support and guidance for academic and professional development, and 3) they play a role in your personal development.

Whichever way you go about identifying potential supervisors, be systematic in your approach to learning about their interests. Your goals should align with theirs. One approach to begin evaluating fit is to create a list of potential supervisors, noting their academic affiliation(s), department(s), and, of course, specific areas of interest. Speak to colleagues or mentors who have worked with these potential supervisors to get different perspectives. After creating your list of serious contenders, the next step is to meet with them. A common method of initiating those meetings is to send an email explaining who you are, your educational and research background, and your areas of interest, highlighting how they align with those of the researcher. The objective of your email is to set up a meeting to discuss the possibility of them supervising your doctoral research. Below is an example of general template that may be used to initiate contact:

Dear Professor X,

I am a [second-year] MD-PhD student interested in studying [X] as part of my doctoral research. [Explain how you came to know about Professor X, their research, and their lab]. [Explain a bit about your research background].

I would be interested in meeting with you to discuss the possibility of conducting my doctoral studies under your supervision. Please let me know whether you would be open to supervising my research and whether you are available for a meeting in the next few weeks.

Best wishes,

[Your name]

This structure is ideal as it is to the point, provides a brief introduction to you, shows your interest and how you came to know about the professor and their work (beyond just seeing their name on the department website), and ends with a request for a face-to-face meeting to discuss PhD research supervision. If they are interested in meeting with you, prepare for the meeting as though it is an interview, since it is. Importantly, recognize this is a two-way interview: they are interviewing you for a position as their PhD student, and you are also interviewing them for the position as your PhD supervisor.

Ahead of the meeting, prepare the questions you would like to discuss with them. Your discussion will likely begin with rearticulating your research interests and thoughts on how they fit with your potential supervisor's research program. Relevant questions to ask and consider include details about what researchers in their lab are currently working on and the direction of future research. Asking specific questions about what their expectations are for their PhD students allows you to determine whether you are on the same page. Here are some other questions you might want to ask:

- Have you previously supervised an MD-PhD student?
- How would you describe your supervisory style?
- What are your thoughts/expectations regarding my timeline as an MD-PhD student?

- Do you have funding to support [describe the project(s) you are interested in conducting]?
- Will I be expected to apply for additional scholarships or grants to fund my research (perhaps in addition to stipends you are already receiving from your MD-PhD program)?

ASSESSING THE DYNAMICS OF YOUR POTENTIAL RESEARCH GROUP

Just as important as the dynamic with your supervisor are the dynamics among the lab members or research group. Current students will have the best insight into the functioning of the lab and the interactions between members. Ask them about how supportive the research group is and whether they would choose the research group again if given the opportunity.

Speak to master's students, PhD students, and postdoctoral researchers, but note that the expectations may be different at different training levels. Speak to lab technicians and lab managers as well. However, you are likely to obtain the most accurate picture of what to expect as a doctoral student in the lab by speaking to current or former doctoral students. Ask the supervisor to put you in contact with a current and/or former student. Students will often give honest answers, especially if the conversations are had in person, as opposed to via email. Ask current and former students about different aspects of their experiences, including what it was like to be a member of the research group, the culture and work practices of the lab, and opportunities to meet with or get feedback from the supervisor. Consider asking about whether lab members work collaboratively or alone, whether lab members arrive and leave at certain hours, or whether everyone follows their own daily schedule. Prepare a list of any questions that you may have for the lab members. Questions you may consider asking current or former students are:

- What made you decide on this particular supervisor?
- How long do students take on average to finish their PhD under this supervisor?
- How do you account for that timeline?
- What are the strengths and weaknesses of the supervisor?
- How much guidance and support were you provided with?
- How frequently did the supervisor meet with you and follow your progress?
- What are the dynamics like between lab members and the supervisor?
- Do they have a network of collaborators that they reach out to to leverage other expertise?

A great way to get a sense of how members of the lab or research group interact with one another and with the supervisor is to attend lab meetings. Meetings where members of the research team present their work or other relevant research often elicit a lot of discussion among the team. The richness of discussion, feedback, and the tone that members use can be an important way to gauge how the research team works and interacts. When you are visiting the research group, consider different aspects of the research environment: Is the lab a size that will work well for you? What is the general atmosphere? Do people seem happy?

The importance of the last question cannot be understated. An indelible memory: in one research group meeting, a very accomplished and productive postdoctoral researcher was presenting a progress update on his project. Toward the end of the hour-long meeting, he began to cry while still fielding questions and responding to feedback from the other lab members. Although there may have been other factors in his life that contributed to his reaction, the lack of compassion from his colleagues was striking. Perhaps his research environment was one that allowed him to be maximally productive. In some research groups, the support network is there and is nurtured and valued, and in others, it is not. One way is not necessarily correct or incorrect, but understanding what your needs are as a researcher is important for your success. You will discover, or have already learned, the kinds of environments in which you are likely to thrive. It's worth mentioning that the nature of research group meetings can vary dramatically depending on the group. A useful way to understand the dynamics of the supervisor and research group is to do a research rotation in that lab, which was described in Chapter 9.

A final and important consideration is the department or graduate program in which you will be completing your training. It is worthwhile to meet with the graduate program director or coordinator. Ask about administrative support, course requirements, and the process for your comprehensive/candidacy/qualifying exam (there are many terms used to describe the examination usually taken in the first or second year of doctoral studies to determine whether or not you progress in the program from a doctoral student to a doctoral candidate).

THE SUPERVISOR-STUDENT RELATIONSHIP

Decades ago, the supervisor-student relationship was primarily an authoritarian one. The professor directed the student and the student's role was to follow the direction of the professor. That relationship has evolved; however, many supervisors may still be accustomed to this model because that was the nature of their relationship with their PhD supervisor. In most research environments today, supervisors still have some authority, but it is recognized that they are not the only source of knowledge. The expertise, open-mindedness, and creativity of students are increasingly respected. Moreover, supervisors are realizing that PhD graduates are navigating and carving out careers that are different from their own. Hence, they are no longer establishing relationships with students based on the idea that the student is meant to follow the supervisor's path. PhD students are expected to be more independent, developing and pursuing many of their own ideas. The role of the supervisor is to oversee this work, ensure it is meeting the expectations of the PhD training program, and provide support and access to resources that allow the student to achieve their goals. The supervisor and the student, however, are both responsible for the outcomes of the student's work (publications, presentations, and the thesis).

The main ingredients that support a healthy relationship between the student and supervisor include mutual respect; resources to support the student's training; and communication channels for advice, encouragement, and the discussion of progress, successes, and challenges. There are different approaches to combining these ingredients, but they should all be present for the relationship to be healthy.

Some students may need more support and structure to reach their goals; Other students may be better suited to a supervisor providing support and encouragement but less structure. The laissez-faire, hands-off supervisory approach is best for a student who doesn't need regular meetings, input or follow-ups to achieve their goals, one who works best in a less structured environment where timelines are flexible and the supervisor does not impose deadlines to advance the work. The old approach to PhD supervision, where the supervisor provides a lot of structure (e.g. specific instructions, tasks and deadlines) but less support and encouragement may work for some students who do not feel they need much external validation; however, it is difficult for many students to thrive long-term without feeling supported.

Overall, independence as a researcher is an important skill to develop and strengthen during your PhD, but you want to avoid a supervisor who creates delays by not being available for meetings or being too busy to review work and provide feedback.

SINGLE VERSUS CO-SUPERVISION

Many PhD students are supervised by a single professor who primarily follows their progress of a student. In this case it is easier to figure out the dynamics of the student and supervisor and the supervision style. However, co-supervision is increasingly common, as many PhD students are working on projects that are interdisciplinary or go beyond the expertise of a single researcher.

Having more than one supervisor can provide additional insights and guidance on your research. Typically, the most co-supervisors one may have is two. There are a few things to think about before embarking on the co-supervision approach. First, it is helpful to know about the potential supervisors' work history. Consider, for example, whether they have co-supervised a student together before, their shared publications, and grant-writing history. How collaborative are they, and how successful are their collaborations? You should also be aware of the benefits and challenges of co-supervision.

Benefits of co-supervision

Some of the benefits include the added perspective that another expert in the field can bring to your project. It even allows you to work with someone who may not be at your institution but is a great source of guidance and direction throughout your PhD. You also benefit from having more connections and networking opportunities. This may be valuable for collaborations during your doctoral research, but also for mentorship, postdoctoral, or academic positions. Your co-supervisor may help to open additional doors that provide you with opportunities to guest lecture, write book chapters, or be involved in other aspects of academic and professional development. The co-supervision model tends to work particularly well when both supervisors have a good working relationship with one another.

Challenges of co-supervision

It sometimes happens that co-supervisors get into disagreements about aspects of your research. Although these disagreements can lead to rich discussions and new directions in your work, they can also slow you down. You will likely take on the role of a mediator in this type of situation, which can be an additional source of stress. This can become problematic if co-supervisors cannot agree at all. Hence, it is important to know about their work history before committing to this type of arrangement with two potential supervisors. It is also a good idea to prepare a document outlining the expectations between you and your supervisors. This document should be very concrete and practical. For instance, if you need documents to be reviewed, who will you send them to first? It might not always be your primary supervisor, especially if your co-supervisor is quicker to respond or is more involved in a particular aspect of your project. A clear, shared understanding among everyone involved is a good starting point for navigating co-supervision.

Often, your primary supervisor will be more up-to-date on your projects and progress. As the PhD student, it is your responsibility to update your co-supervisor about the advancements of your project, through meetings (in person or videoconference), email, or other means.

SUPPORT IN PURSUING YOUR PROJECT AND LARGER CAREER GOALS

Maybe you have an idea of what you want your project to be. You might have even prepared a research proposal outlining this project as part of your MD-PhD application. The reality is that the topic and direction of your proposed research will likely change over the course of your training. Defining your project is a later process, addressed in Chapter 11. It is not realistic to make your decision about a supervisor or research group based solely on the expectation of doing a specific project. There are many other factors to consider, especially time constraints. This is where flexibility and adaptability become key. Although you are on a tighter timeline than the average PhD student, the expectations placed on you in terms of rigor and contributions are the same as any other PhD student. Choosing a research group and supervisor that will support you in achieving this goal is paramount. It will benefit you greatly to discuss your timeline with your potential supervisor as early as possible and adjust your expectations about your project, if necessary.

As a doctoral student, you are still viewed as a trainee; however, as you advance in your area of research, you will develop an expertise. It is valuable to your development as a researcher if your supervisor recognizes this expertise as you progress. Consult with previous students and ask about how their dynamic with their supervisor changed as they advanced in their studies. Did the supervisor adjust their expectations of the student over time? It often takes time to integrate into a new research environment and learn the practices of the lab before a PhD student can be independent and productive. Ask current students if they feel they have independence. Are they comfortable with the amount of direction the supervisor provides? This balance may vary for different students. Obtaining perspectives from different students can help you to decide whether you'll receive the support you need to finish your PhD research. Your supervisor should be available to meet with you and discuss your progress at a frequency that meets your needs.

An important measure of productivity during doctoral studies is publications, conference presentations, and successful scholarships and grants. Current and former students will be able to share with you whether the supervisor provided them with opportunities to publish their work, present at conferences, apply for awards, and be a coinvestigator on research grants. These types of opportunities will be important to open doors for a future career in academia. Applications for postdoctoral fellowships and faculty positions will consider your publication list, participation in conferences and meetings, as well as funding that you were able to secure to advance your research projects. Your supervisor plays an important role in positioning you for future success as an independent investigator.

Your career goals may not be the same as your supervisor's, and that is okay. Supervisors should not impose their career goals on you, but they can still be a valuable source of mentorship and support. Ideally, the student-supervisor relationship that one establishes during the PhD will continue after you have defended and submitted your thesis. Your supervisor can support you in achieving your larger career goals even after you have left their lab.

CONCLUSION

The research group and supervisor that you choose will be your village for the next few years. The decision is important and highly personal. It is informed by much more than just the research project. Within the structure of most MD-PhD programs, you have time to make this important decision. Take advantage of this time to reflect on what you want out of the experience and what you need to help you achieve those goals. Use the time that you have before starting your PhD to explore your options. The process itself is also an opportunity to learn about yourself and how other researchers and research groups function—information that may be valuable to you as an independent researcher with your own research group. Landing in a supportive village can make a huge difference during your PhD and position you for success afterward.

Part III

The Transition to Graduate School

11

Defining Your Project

Jared Hinkle • Chirag Vasavda

Jared Hinkle *entered the MD-PhD program at Johns Hopkins University in 2015 and joined the Department of Neuroscience graduate program in 2017. He is conducting his PhD thesis research in the laboratories of Drs. Ted and Valina Dawson and is currently investigating how glial cells respond to fibrillar α-synuclein in Parkinson disease.*

Chirag Vasavda *entered the MD-PhD program at Johns Hopkins University in 2014. He joined the Biochemistry, Cellular and Molecular Biology graduate program and studied under Dr. Solomon Snyder in the Department of Neuroscience. In graduate school, he discovered that the heme metabolite bilirubin binds and activates the orphan receptor MRGPRX4 in itch sensory neurons, potentially contributing to itch in hepatobiliary disease. He also identified that bilirubin is a physiologic antioxidant with distinct redox activity that negatively regulates superoxide signaling during neurotransmission.*

INTRODUCTION

In order to complete the PhD phase of your training, you will need to conduct a systematic research study under the guidance of the principal investigator (PI) of your research lab. Students identify a PI through their research rotations, as discussed in Chapter 9, and make the official decision to join a PI's laboratory or research group sometime early in the PhD

> **WHAT YOU NEED TO KNOW**
>
> - PhD projects are defined in close collaboration with your PI through an iterative process, typically over the first 3–12 months after joining the lab. However, a PhD thesis is never completely defined until it is in fact complete—it is an evolutionary process with stages of stability and periods of revision.
> - Topically and methodologically, PhD projects tend to fall close to the core interests of the laboratory head and previous work the lab has done. However, there is no formulaic one-size-fits-all approach for PIs and graduate students in defining a project.
> - Preliminary data are essential to demonstrating the plausibility of your hypotheses and will likely become integrated into your proposal for thesis work.
> - A combination of high-risk-high-reward and more easily achieved projects is often ideal.
> - Your thesis committee will help you to shape the thesis project as you progress and ultimately decide when your research is sufficient to earn the PhD degree.

program. Unlike the predefined coursework of the preclinical medical school curriculum or core graduate school coursework, the PhD thesis project is not a curated experience. Rather, each student works with their PI to identify the topic of the thesis research project and to articulate a strategy for the investigation. This chapter addresses the nature of this process, its relationship to your scientific training, and some general guidelines for successfully identifying a feasible PhD project.

AN EVER-CHANGING TIMELINE

While completing research rotations, MD-PhD students learn about the kind of investigations they might conduct in the lab and will most likely discuss project ideas with prospective mentors. Once the decision to join a laboratory or research group has been made, the process of defining a research project for PhD training can commence in full. In many PhD programs, students are expected to create—with the PI's guidance—a thesis proposal that articulates the scientific background, hypotheses, methodological approach, and preliminary evidence for the thesis project. This proposal may be tied to the process of becoming a full-fledged PhD candidate, as its completion signals that the student and PI have a plan of action for PhD training over the next several years. Ultimately, this work is expected to culminate in the student's dissertation, thesis defense, and peer-reviewed manuscript(s).

It is typical to describe PhD training with the sort of sequential or stage-based overview expressed earlier in this chapter. While this is useful for understanding the general timeline and the expectations for graduation, it can belie the complexity of defining the specific scientific content of PhD training. Early in training, you may have the opportunity to see finalized PhD thesis projects that were completed by others before you. From this perspective, the PhD thesis project can appear to be a generally coherent process. However, it is important to recognize early on that this is usually not the case—PhD projects are evolutionary by nature. While some projects come together quickly, many can take time to mature into something that will resemble the final product. The same may be said of the peer-reviewed publications with which you will engage intensively throughout the PhD. It's important to mentally separate your works in progress from the polished final products that appear in publications and research talks.

DEFINING SHORT-TERM AND LONG-TERM GOALS

Having acknowledged the messy reality of day-to-day science and the convoluted nature of many research projects, there are plenty of practical steps that you can take to define a project that is likely to be successful and to accelerate your growth as a scientist. More details on maximizing research productivity throughout your studies can be found in Chapter 12, while the advice included here should be especially useful from the very start of your project. For example, a trainee should consider how their project goals and ideas mesh with the interests and expertise of the laboratory environment. If you are proposing to employ methods that are not regularly used in the lab, it is important to be cognizant of how this could affect the time required to make progress. Heuristically, PhD projects tend to fall more closely within the established research domain of the PI, whereas postdoctoral researchers may leverage their experience to effectively push into new areas. Various circumstances may lead a PhD candidate to explore new methodological avenues, such as a collaboration with another lab or a "co-PI" thesis project. In this case, it is particularly important that the student and primary PI have a shared sense of purpose and interests. The laboratory head is responsible for ensuring that their students develop as scientists, which includes guiding the choice of research topic in an appropriate direction. Therefore, clear communication of goals and expectations is essential to identifying a project that will ultimately be successful with respect to the quality of scientific training and the productivity of the PhD.

While defining your thesis project, it can be extremely helpful to think about it as a long-term career development initiative. In other words, you might consider the future self as a part of scientific productivity during the PhD phase. Graduate programs are using taxpayer dollars to enable your acquisition of expertise and intellectual advancement as scientist and scholar, so try to think about how performing this project will help justify that support. For example, what specific skills will you acquire and how do they relate to your long-term career objectives? Are there alternative or additional strategies or research aims you could consider that would enhance your training? Will the scientific or biomedical topics related to this research be important in the coming decades? These are difficult questions. It is therefore important to seek out advice from not only your PI, but also fellow graduate students, mentors, and other colleagues when considering the answers. They will take some time to work through, and there may be a bit of instability or indecision in the beginning stages of your project, which is normal.

COLLECTING DATA WHILE STAYING FLEXIBLE

As you work on defining your project, you will concurrently be learning techniques and using them to test your hypotheses, thereby (hopefully) generating *preliminary data*. These are data that may not represent a complete story and are not necessarily "publication quality." Rather, they are used to show the feasibility of your project and assess the likelihood that your hypotheses are correct. These may include evidence of phenomena that are necessary but not sufficient for your hypothesis to be correct. For example, suppose you are ultimately interested in knowing whether a signaling pathway is hyperactivated in a specific cell type in a given disease state. You might first test whether an element of this pathway is upregulated at the protein or mRNA level in vitro using cells from the disease model. This upregulation might be necessary for the pathway to be active, but not sufficient. Similarly, preliminary data often lacks the comprehensive specificity that a final publication typically has. For example, if the element you are examining can be upregulated by multiple upstream signaling pathways, then it might be the case that a different pathway is responsible for the upregulation you observe. Ultimately, you may need to produce genetically altered cell lines or model organisms to test this hypothesis more specifically, but in the meantime, your preliminary data will serve as the justification for these long-term objectives. These examples illustrate the limited interpretability that is typical of preliminary data but illustrates how they are ultimately helpful for showing the plausibility of your ideas.

Remember, you will be spending at least 2–3 years working on your PhD project, so it is important not to get too invested in a particular hypothesis or narrative without having at least some indication that your project will bear fruit. On the other hand, exploratory or descriptive modes of science may set different expectations for what constitutes preliminary data. For example, your project might involve generating large amounts of transcriptomic data and seeing what patterns emerge from them. While it is still important to have a clear set of rationales or goals for such investigations, it may be less critical to have a highly specific hypothesis with individual units of evidence. In this case, preliminary evidence might be some observation supporting the plausibility of your experimental approach, such as a validation of sequencing data. Finally, it is not uncommon for PhD projects to be extensions of prior or existing projects conducted by others in the laboratory. In this case, preliminary evidence might derive from or build upon the observations of other lab members. For example, it is not uncommon for a thesis proposal to include—with appropriate attribution—data that were obtained by or with the assistance of an older graduate student or a postdoctoral researcher.

One question that might arise during PhD training is *how many* projects to be pursuing at once. Having at least one side project can carry some potential benefits, depending on how you strategize. For example, if your main project breaks down at some point, then you have a fallback plan. Even if the main project doesn't become untenable, side projects may help you fill the time between experiments and acquire some useful skills in the process. You might also choose a high-risk-high-reward endeavor as a side project. If this starts to become promising, you could then shift attention to it, but if it doesn't work out, you still have your principal project for thesis and publication purposes. However, it is important to avoid a scenario where you have spread yourself too thin between multiple projects. Similarly, it can be problematic to assume a mindset where you are more focused on coming up with new projects than with finishing what you already have on your plate. While this may be satisfying in the short term, it can make it difficult to generate a compelling and focused narrative for your thesis. Inefficiencies can also arise in this context due to task-switching if the projects involve very different bodies of background literature to keep up with or experimental approaches to master. However, if you can define a side project that does not overly tax your attention or distract from your core thesis work, it may be worth discussing with your PI. It can also be ideal to share some of the groundwork for a side project with another lab member, especially if they have the methodological experience to help you efficiently obtain some preliminary data.

GETTING TO WORK WITH YOUR THESIS COMMITTEE

Once you have settled into a particular project area (i.e., you have generated some preliminary data and have a good idea of your thesis proposal), it is time to get to work! As you begin to make progress on the work outlined in your project, some experiments may yield data more readily than others, and some techniques may pose more difficulties than others. It is essential to know how to ask for help in interpreting your data, especially early on in this process.

In addition to your fellow lab members, you will also have the guidance of a thesis committee throughout your PhD training. This is a small group of two to four faculty—in addition to your PI—who will assess your progress as a scientist and the quality of your research project as it evolves. Most PhD programs require formal thesis committee meetings once or twice a year, depending on how the committee thinks you are doing (i.e., the committee may deem it acceptable to assemble less frequently if the project is going exceptionally smoothly). The main purpose of these meetings is to ensure that you are meeting the benchmarks of PhD training; thus, these meetings serve as opportunities to get feedback on your work and advice for clearing unexpected hurdles. It is not uncommon for a thesis committee to notice exciting alternative directions for a PhD student to pursue or to identify previously unnoticed problems with how the data are being interpreted. The committee members are there to help you advance your research and also serve as additional expert eyes on the oversight afforded by your PI. Therefore, it can be highly beneficial to take full advantage of these meetings early and regularly get fresh insights and energizing ideas.

The thesis committee is also largely responsible for confirming when your project is complete—that is, when you can defend your thesis and graduate—so it is certainly worth putting your best foot forward in these meetings. Viewing them as opportunities for formative feedback and guidance—rather than only critical assessment—can work wonders for your project's significance. It is also not uncommon for thesis committee members to raise opportunities for experimental collaborations, which can forge new relationships and generate exciting data.

CONCLUSION

Your thesis project will most likely be one of the most intellectually challenging phases of your career as an MD-PhD student, but hopefully also one of the most meaningful and formative. Proactively seeking guidance from your PI and other mentors at the beginning phases of your project will help to maximize the eventual payoff. Similarly, being critical of your early preliminary data and considering multiple interpretations will help define the early direction of your project and the ultimate shape of your thesis narrative. Chapters 15 and 16 ("Completing Your Project" and "Thesis Writing," respectively) contain advice on how to integrate your research into an excellent thesis. Ultimately, however, remember that your thesis is an expression of your unique thinking style, your laboratory's environment and technical approach, and the scientific questions that compel you. Therefore, there is no formulaic approach to getting a PhD or to completing a thesis. This reality can and will be alternately confusing, daunting, and exhilarating. Do not hesitate to lean on fellows and senior graduate students for advice. It can be hard trying to navigate the emotional turbulence of your thesis project while staying focused on the big picture. Most importantly, have fun!

12

Maximizing Research Productivity

Shriya Deshmukh

Shriya Deshmukh *is a fifth-year MD-PhD student at McGill University. Her PhD research is in experimental medicine and centers on uncovering epigenetic mechanisms driving the development of pediatric high-grade gliomas and neurodevelopmental syndromes. Prior to medical school, Shriya completed a bachelor of science in neuroscience from the University of Toronto.*

INTRODUCTION

This chapter focuses on insights into maximizing research productivity as an MD-PhD student. Unlike other graduate students, MD-PhD students typically have restrictions on the time they can devote to graduate studies, as imposed by program structure and the demands of concurrently completing a medical degree. In addition, because most MD-PhDs pursue clinical residencies upon graduation, there is a considerable gap between the conclusion of graduate studies and the start of their careers as physician-scientists. Research techniques, technologies, and knowledge progress at a rate considerably faster than the training trajectory of physician-scientists. Moreover, it is probable that research interests will diverge with the acquisition of additional clinical experiences during residency. Therefore, in this chapter, we focus on research skills that will serve MD-PhD graduates well even after a hiatus of several years.

As a student in the fourth year of my PhD, I am acutely aware of the time constraints of my graduate research program. Working in Dr. Nada Jabado's lab, I study the epigenome's role in the development of aggressive high-grade pediatric brain tumors and other cancers using

---

WHAT YOU NEED TO KNOW

- Attend conferences and scientific meetings to learn, receive feedback, network with collaborators, and refocus your own projects.
- Find a simple and effortless way to keep up-to-date with new research in your field: email alerts, social media, local meetings, journal clubs, etc.
- Take student supervision responsibilities seriously.
- Use committee meetings to assess progress and develop plans to achieve your goals.
- Through uncertainty and failure, be open and seek help when necessary. Remind yourself why you love doing research!

various next-generation sequencing technologies, gene editing, and functional assays. The lab consists of a diverse, talented, and close-knit group of individuals, and we frequently interact with local and international collaborators across a spectrum of research and clinical disciplines. My time spent in this fun, fast-paced, and intellectually stimulating environment has taught me the importance of taking purposeful steps to promote research productivity.

Research productivity can be narrowly defined in terms of the number and quality of publications produced; this topic is covered at length in the following chapter. In this chapter, we take an expansive view of research productivity to encompass the development of foundational skills that will promote future research productivity. This chapter includes insights into presenting at conferences, keeping up-to-date with novel research findings, and taking advantage of committee meetings and exams to propel your projects forward.

EFFECTIVE COMMUNICATION IS ESSENTIAL

Effective communication is a foundational skill that is key to producing effective research. Effective communication enables audiences to understand your research and the importance of your findings. Clear communication is as important for fellow scientists seeking to evaluate the veracity of your claims as for a lay audience trying to grasp the implications of your research. If audiences can clearly understand your research, this translates into them being able to provide more insightful feedback.

Not only is clear communication important for others, it is also helpful for organizing your own ideas. The process of developing a cohesive and coherent narrative centered on your research findings can lead you to develop novel insights into your own research. The time devoted to explaining your results to others can help you to better interpret the data and develop ideas for follow-up experiments. It can also highlight flaws in experimental design or problematic analyses that may have been overlooked during the data generation process.

Persuasive writing is especially important to securing grants that will enable you to test hypotheses and execute your research plan. To support your research goals, you need to provide a compelling case to funding agencies on the feasibility and value of your research. See Chapter 17 for further insights on the value of communication and networking in your search for grants and scholarships.

Science today is rarely conducted in isolation. Instead, collaboration is the norm. To build a team of individuals with different expertise working toward a common goal, you need to be able to communicate effectively with everyone. This is especially pertinent for MD-PhD students and graduates, since they straddle research and clinical fields and have a responsibility to bridge the divide between scientists and clinicians, promoting tangible improvements in patient health.

CONFERENCES AND MEETINGS

Conferences can be a great way to learn about new discoveries from leading scientists in your field. They are also opportunities to share your research, receive feedback, and develop new ideas for your projects. Take care, however, to strike a balance between attending useful conferences and working on your research projects. Considering the time constraints for MD-PhD students, it is important that you submit abstracts judiciously, taking into account the impact that travel and time away from the lab will have on your research progress. A dozen abstracts and presentations at various conferences will not substitute for an impactful paper.

Selecting the right conference

How then do you choose which conferences to attend? As MD-PhD students, you have a unique perspective on clinical and scientific questions and may be interested in attending both clinical and basic/translational science-intensive conferences. Attending diverse conferences will enable you to build a network with people of different expertise. It may also strengthen different aspects of your research upon receiving feedback from different sources. If your supervisor does not have a clinical background or attend clinical conferences, you may want to discuss the possibility of attending clinical conferences to help you develop clinically relevant projects for your thesis.

Striking a balance between attending local, national, and international conferences is also important. Prior to or at the start of your graduate studies, speak with your supervisor and other lab members to get a sense of conferences that they recommend and are well-attended by the lab. Seek to attend these conferences at least once during your graduate training. Try then to balance local with national and international conferences, where participants and speakers will vary considerably.

Above all, attend conferences that will spark new ideas about your own projects. For this reason, although it may be enticing to attend large conferences that draw reputed scientists and showcase a wide range of research subjects, these conferences ultimately may not be useful venues for developing and progressing your own research aims. Smaller, more focused meetings can present excellent opportunities to learn about new discoveries in your field, interact with key leaders, and receive specific feedback on your research from experts in your field of interest. Smaller conferences also often have allotted free time to encourage group activities and interactions among participants. Take advantage of this time by organizing informal meetings with collaborators with whom you may previously only have interacted by teleconference. In-person meetings are usually more productive and are fantastic opportunities to share new data and ideas, discuss project timelines, and develop stronger relationships.

Take a break and enjoy time away from the lab!

Remember that after the conference you want to come back to your research with fresh ideas, feeling rejuvenated. It can be easy to feel diminished and daunted at conferences, both by the expectation that you need to attend every lecture and event, and by the sheer amount of new research presented. Take a break when you need to. There's no point trying to focus on the minutiae of a dense scientific talk through bleary eyes or rushing through every poster starred on your list. Sometimes the most productive thing can be to relax and try a nonscience activity with fellow conference participants. Seasoned conference-goers will tell you that some of the most interesting scientific ideas are shared and developed in informal settings during informal conversations.

Useful meetings

Conferences are not the only venues to interact with members of the scientific community. Your supervisor may be involved in group initiatives and collaborations with focused research aims. If your supervisor is coinvestigator on a program project grant or large-scale research project with ties to your projects, you may want to ask to be involved in meetings to learn about relevant research and to interact with collaborators.

For instance, my PI is coinvestigator on a National Institutes of Health (NIH) P01 Research Program Project Grant. Although we interact regularly with collaborators that are part of this grant, I find the in-person annual meetings to be an excellent way to learn new information from and interact effectively with our collaborators. Discussions and ideas flow faster, collaborations are more easily established, and non-meeting activities break the ice more effectively. In the process, you also gain fascinating insights into the organization and management of large-scale collaborative scientific projects.

Perfecting presentation skills

Finally, you may be wondering why this section focuses so little on the actual process of writing abstracts and preparing oral and poster presentations. This is because, after acquiring the basic structure for writing abstracts and preparing poster and oral presentations (for which there are many available resources), each budding scientist needs to follow a trial-and-error process to find the style that works best for them. Effective presenters that I can remember have spoken fast or slow, taken 10 seconds or 10 minutes per slide, used analogies to explain research findings or not, delved into or skimmed through complex figures and graphs, amongst many other contradictions. What they invariably shared was a visible enthusiasm for sharing their research findings, data presented that centered around a clear central message targeted to the audience, and a logical progression in their presentation. This is obviously easier said than done, and I continue to work on my own presentation skills with the guidance of my PI and colleagues. Chapter 17, on networking as an MD-PhD student, contains useful tips and strategies for preparing effective presentations.

KEEPING UP-TO-DATE

One of the most difficult aspects of research in the twenty-first century is becoming accustomed to the pace of new discoveries and the deluge of daily new publications. It can be especially difficult to maintain the motivation to keep updated with new discoveries in your field of interest when you are immersed in conducting experiments; performing analyses; or writing grants, papers, and reports. However, neglecting to take the time to know where your field has progressed and is headed can have significant costs. This section provides some tips that can facilitate this task and help to develop a manageable routine.

Take advantage of "dead" time

My favorite resource is the automatic My NCBI email alert for keyword searches. Instead of regularly searching PubMed for keywords relevant to your research project or discipline to find new papers, you can create a My NCBI account and set up email alerts specific to certain keyword searches. The settings can be personalized; I like to read abstracts (not just titles of papers) and have set up different alert schedules (daily versus weekly) for different keywords. These short email alerts are excellent, because they can be read during "dead" time, while waiting in line or during the daily commute. Papers that seem relevant and important can be bookmarked to be read later. Similarly, subscribing to email alerts for tables of contents from journals of interest can be useful. Summaries or editorial commentaries on relevant or interesting journal articles can be quickly perused during "dead" time as well.

Social media: To do or not to do?

Social media can be a time sink and distraction. However, social media is also increasingly being harnessed by scientists to share new discoveries and ideas amongst themselves and with the wider community. Following key scientific communicators on platforms such as Twitter can be a simple way to learn about exciting research being conducted, science policy, education challenges, advice to young scientists, and ethical debates. Many journals also maintain a presence on social media platforms like Facebook, enabling easy browsing of editorial commentary on key articles.

Numerous online resources are also available to connect you with different scientific communities. For example, Slack is a website designed to facilitate team communication through various messaging and file-sharing tools. Many graduate students and scientists use Slack to connect with each other and share ideas and advice on any number of topics: research field-specific topics (e.g., bioinformatics, molecular genomics), preparing for qualifying exams, drafting papers/theses, professional and career growth, and job opportunities. This online community can be particularly useful when you are unable to find the necessary resources in your lab or university locally.

Participate in the local research community

In addition to attending conferences to keep up-to-date with your field, joining and participating in local research groups or journal clubs is an excellent way to learn about new research techniques, methodologies, and discoveries. For instance, I participated in a monthly seminar series initiated by a postdoctoral fellow, which brings together students and scientists from different institutions in Montreal (e.g., Rosalind and Morris Goodman Cancer Research Centre, The Research Institute of the McGill University Health Centre, Centre hospitalier de l'université de Montreal) with a common interest in functional genomics. Not only do these seminars provide a wide perspective on different kinds of research, they also serve as useful networking opportunities: You can form new local collaborations and seek advice on your own projects. Moreover, there may be times as a graduate student when your projects fail to excite you and your experiments become routine and monotonous. Attending these local gatherings can animate you once more about your research, stimulate new ideas, and gather some energy from the social support of fellow graduate students. Finally, if these research groups don't exist in your local environment, create them yourself! Consult with your supervisor, colleagues, graduate department, or research institute about the need to establish a new group, and request their help in securing a venue and advertising to relevant individuals.

SUPERVISING STUDENTS

As you become established in the lab, you may be tasked with the responsibility of supervising one or more students, whether undergraduates, junior graduate students, or medical students. This can be a surprisingly challenging task, even when you are supervising the most motivated students. It can take time away from your experiments, analyses, and writing to closely supervise a student and ensure their daily progress. However, the sense of reward and pride that comes from observing your student's development and growth is enormous. It is also a necessary skill for both clinicians and scientists to learn to teach others.

Present and discuss options

It's important to set the framework early for your relationship with your student. Have a frank discussion about their time commitment, project interests, and expectations, as well as your own. In my experience, it's unusual for students to have a clear idea of which projects they would like to work on; instead, these discussions usually focus on skills or experimental techniques they wish to acquire. It's important to explain the projects that are ongoing and allow some opportunity for students to explore different experimental techniques. I think this is especially important for students with limited time in the lab, such as summer students. The kinds of projects we work on in a basic science wet lab rarely produce results within the two-month time frame of a summer studentship. Although it's important for students to understand that failure is a part of science, it can be dispiriting for them to concentrate solely on one project, only to see it fail. That is why learning and trying different experimental techniques over the course of the summer, while working on their own projects, can be a better option.

Enable and encourage student ownership and participation in research

Always ensure that your student has ownership over their project. Their project can be a small part of a much bigger project, but it is essential that your student feel ownership over their work, rather than someone called upon to do a little for dozens of projects. Encourage your student to independently read papers and develop ideas, experiments, and protocols to advance their project. Include them in project discussions and meetings with collaborators so that they understand the broader scope of the project. Try to encourage their participation in lab meeting presentations and student research days, and always acknowledge their contribution to your projects. Reward their initiative with your attention and support. Be patient and kind with failures: of the many undergraduate students who have worked in our lab, all have been well-intentioned, and all took their failed experiments much more personally than us seasoned graduate students, who recognize failure as par for the course.

You may be wondering what these supervisory strategies have to do with your research productivity. The simple answer is that by ensuring your student's success, you effectively ensure your own. The more productive your student is, the further your projects advance. Furthermore, as your student develops, you may be surprised by their insights and innovative ideas. And if that doesn't seem enough, remember that we've all had incredible mentors who took the time to teach us and supported our goals and aspirations; it's simply time to pay it forward.

GRADUATE COURSES

Graduate course requirements vary considerably by department. However, given the limited time frame of your graduate studies, if you have the option of selecting between multiple graduate departments, consider applying to one with less onerous coursework requirements. The best advisors are senior graduate and MD-PhD students who can provide candid opinions about the strengths of various departments with respect to coursework and available administrative support. The administrative resources of a department may seem like a trivial matter to inquire about but can significantly impact processes ranging from scheduling committee meetings to submitting scholarship applications. Larger departments often have more resources; better designed, more transparent requirements; and more support for graduate students.

Once you know the coursework requirements specified by your department, try to complete the required courses as soon as possible. Doing so will not only provide you with the necessary foundation to develop your research projects early but will also enable you to focus more time on completing your projects, papers, and thesis toward the end of your graduate program.

Selecting graduate courses

Some departments specify mandatory introductory-level courses. Once these are completed, there is typically a significant degree of flexibility in your choice of subsequent courses. It's important to consult with your supervisor, since they may have course recommendations that would benefit your research. Similarly, discussing with fellow graduate students in your lab can help you to decide on useful and relevant courses (as well as avoiding others). Graduate courses can also be a great way to expand your knowledge on a subject area outside your research field. For instance, I decided to take a newly offered graduate course on artificial intelligence because I wanted to learn more about its applications in medicine. Although what I learned in this course wasn't immediately relevant to my research, I enjoyed the challenge of learning something new. I also recommend taking scientific and persuasive writing courses. Writing well is a skill that will always be important and can always be improved upon.

Lastly, my personal advice to you is to select courses where the subject interests you, and not based on the number of assignments, exams, or grading criteria. We have all suffered through courses where the subject matter was painfully uninteresting to us; given the freedom to choose, choose wisely.

COMMITTEE MEETINGS AND THE COMPREHENSIVE EXAMINATION

Selecting your committee

Most graduate departments require students to have an annual meeting with members of their thesis committee. Choosing committee members is a decision that will likely fall to you and your supervisor. You may be required to choose committee members early in graduate school, before you have had many opportunities to connect with scientists in the local environment. Asking fellow or previous graduate students about the composition of their committees is a good starting point to shortlist candidates. Importantly, consider the support you will require for different aspects of your projects and aim to ask individuals with a diverse set of knowledge and expertise corresponding to your projects. It may also be necessary to change the composition of your committee as your projects evolve and different expertise is required. These decisions should be made in consultation with your supervisor.

Perfecting presentation skills

Guidelines for submitted reports and meeting format will vary across different graduate departments. In general, however, prepare for committee meetings by reading extensively on the research area of your projects. Prepare your presentation well in advance and present to lab members and your supervisor to receive their feedback for improvements. Think back to the presentation techniques that have been successful at conferences and meetings. Two key components to a committee meeting presentation are your research question(s) and hypotheses: many graduate students struggle to articulate these clearly and can leave the committee confused during the rest of the presentation as they struggle to associate the experimental plan with the expressed project aims. Spend time making sure that your presentation is as clear as possible, because this will greatly improve the subsequent discussion with your committee members. Instead of asking for clarifications, they will be better able to target their questions and provide input on the areas that need to be further developed in your project.

Conduct your own review of personal progress and develop future goals

Use committee meeting presentations as an opportunity to assess your own progress (e.g., courses completed, techniques learned, abstract/conference presentations, publications, ongoing drafts/submissions). Committee meetings are also excellent opportunities to set personal goals and update your development plan. What skills and techniques would you like to develop in the short, medium, and long term? What actions will you take to accomplish these goals? Aim to have SMART goals: specific, measurable, achievable, realistic and time-defined. A helpful resource to start building your own plan is Canadian Institutes of Health Research's (CIHR) Individual Development Plan, available online and designed to help researchers actively manage their career trajectory.

It is important to communicate your goals and timeline to your committee members, since they may be unaware of the MD-PhD program structure. Manage their expectations by providing a reminder at every committee meeting of your timeline. This will enable your committee members to provide you with more specific advice on the scope of your projects to ensure that you are able to graduate on time.

The comprehensive exam: Coming to terms with uncertainty

Many graduate programs have a PhD candidacy/comprehensive/qualifying examination, typically held in the second year of the program. This exam is a way for your committee to assess your potential to successfully earn a PhD. Comprehensive examinations are like committee meetings but are usually more formal and structured: the presentation time limit may be strictly enforced, as will the question-and-answer period. Your committee members may test your knowledge on subjects outside your main research focus and assess your critical thinking skills by asking you to consider different experimental approaches or alternative explanations and interpretations of your data. Don't be daunted by this question-and-answer period. Try to think of it as an intellectually stimulating conversation with your committee members rather than an exam. It's also perfectly fine to admit that you don't know the answer to every question; your committee members will intentionally push you to the limits of your knowledge to understand how you handle uncertainty. What is important is to demonstrate how you grapple with questions for which you don't know the answer and to explain your reasoning process clearly. A helpful exercise in preparation for your exam is to anticipate questions that a reviewer may have based on the presented data. As always, practicing beforehand with your supervisor and colleagues is very helpful.

Finally, use the input and insights shared with you during your committee meetings to improve your projects and papers. You are also encouraged to seek help from your committee members outside of committee meetings to further your research projects.

CONCLUSION

I hope you found these insights into maximizing research productivity useful. As you try to conduct research more efficiently and effectively, remember to take a step back every so often and remind yourself why you love doing research. I love being in the lab and working together with my amazing colleagues and supervisor to answer complex research questions. There have also been times when I've felt frustrated or sad about the seemingly widening chasm between my goals and the current state of my research projects. Research is difficult and uncertain work and sometimes, no matter how hard or efficiently you work, your experiments and even entire projects will fail. It's important to realize that this occurs to everyone and your status as an MD-PhD student doesn't preclude you from experiencing failure in the lab. Opening up to your colleagues, whether in the MD-PhD program or your fellow graduate students, can be extremely helpful, because they will almost invariably empathize with your struggles.

Don't hesitate to take breaks from science, whether to pursue extracurricular activities outside the lab, go on a vacation, or just spend time with family and friends. This is often the best way to recharge and maximize research productivity in the lab. Finally, I think one of the best parts about being an MD-PhD student is that we maintain some degree of contact with patients throughout our graduate studies. There is nothing quite so motivating as interacting with patients and family members who are eagerly supporting your research endeavors in the hope for a better future.

13

Publication

Shriya Deshmukh

Shriya Deshmukh *is a fifth-year MD-PhD student at McGill University. Her PhD research is in experimental medicine and centers on uncovering epigenetic mechanisms driving the development of pediatric high-grade gliomas and neurodevelopmental syndromes. Prior to medical school, Shriya completed a bachelor of science in neuroscience from the University of Toronto.*

INTRODUCTION

Articles remain the currency of scientific knowledge transfer. Done right, producing a scientific paper should reflect an iterative process of generating and engaging with data to derive insights central to research questions, as well as clearly communicating key findings to the scientific community. Engaging in a rigorous peer-review process should strengthen research quality. In this chapter, I share my observations on effectively developing projects to culminate successfully in scientific papers. It is especially important for MD-PhD students to learn how to efficiently translate their work into publications within the graduate timespan. I hope this chapter demystifies the process and helps budding physician-scientists embark on successful projects and papers!

BUILD YOUR PAPER ONE STEP AT A TIME

Writing a publication can be likened to building a house: the plans first need to be prepared, followed by laying the foundations, establishing service connections, constructing the framework for walls and floor, followed by finishing touches, and finally, renovations. Throughout, there needs to be effective communication and coordination between the invested parties (owner, architect, builders, etc.) to ensure that the final product is to everybody's satisfaction.

WHAT YOU NEED TO KNOW

- Create an outline with an experimental plan early and update regularly.
- Good organization is half the battle won when writing a paper.
- Aim for clarity in the figures presented and corresponding text.
- Communicate openly and clearly with your team to prevent interpersonal conflicts.
- Edit, edit, and edit again!

1. Do your homework

At the beginning of graduate studies, you will want to establish a strong foundation in the subject of your project by performing a comprehensive review of the scientific literature. Do not neglect to read old papers that may not be available in a digital format and are consequently more difficult to acquire. Taking the time to understand the historical context of your project is important, and you may be surprised by the clinical insights and hypotheses in these papers that are relevant to your project. During this process, you may want to write a review article that will enable you to familiarize yourself with the research domain while gaining experience writing and publishing a paper.

2. Create an outline (early!)

Preparing the plans involves making a draft or outline of the proposed paper early in the process. This may seem impossible: How can you write an outline without knowing the results of your experiments? In fact, the process of writing a simple introduction and articulating central research questions, hypotheses, and an experimental plan can be very useful. Grant proposals are a good starting point for setting this groundwork. Anticipating experimental results and necessary analyses can also help to identify which experiments are integral (versus tangential) to answering the research questions. This can then help you to focus on key experiments and plan to acquire the tools or training to perform experiments and analyses. This outline should be flexible. As you acquire new data that leads you to alter your original hypotheses and experimental plan, update your outline accordingly.

3. Collaborate and organize projects effectively

The foundations will be laid by the experiments themselves, which are specific to research disciplines and should be embarked upon in consultation with your PI and other relevant members. Most projects involve varying degrees of teamwork to perform the necessary experiments to comprehensively answer the research questions. Connecting different expertise and experiments to move projects and publications forward requires good organization. Coordination between members can be facilitated by online file-sharing services like Dropbox and Google Docs. Create a folder for each project and share with key members of the team. Here's a template for files you may want to include in each project folder:

- Useful resources
  - References: list key articles with a few notes relevant to the project. Update regularly!
  - Links to online databases
- Metadata
  - List the location and format of primary data (e.g., whole genome sequencing of sample X stored in format Y on server Z)
- Materials and methods
  - Experiment protocols and data analysis methods
  - Supplementary tables (e.g., antibodies used, relevant clinical details, etc.)
- Presentations, reports, posters
  - Meeting presentations by you and collaborators
  - Committee meeting reports
  - Conference posters
- Figures
  - Figures and figure legends with every revision
    - Update regularly with each new piece of data and analysis

- Manuscript
  - Written drafts of the manuscript
  - Comments/edits by contributing authors
- Other documents
  - Ethics approval
- Peer review

  - Reviewer comments and response
  - Revised manuscript

By organizing the publication beforehand in a manner that facilitates sharing of data, analyses, and ideas among collaborators, you will have laid the foundation for productive teamwork. Moreover, arranging all files in a central location over time will enable everyone to easily access and retrieve information on previous experiments and analyses; this is especially important for projects of long duration or legacy projects involving the introduction of new students working on the project.

4. Display and narrate your findings clearly and with a logical progression

Constructing the framework of a publication concerns the interpretation of experimental results and data, and shaping these into a cohesive narrative. This is a challenging task. You are often so immersed in the creation and details of your project that the results may seem self-evident. Remember that most scientists will scan papers by quickly reading the abstract and glancing at figures and legends before deciding whether to invest into a thorough perusal of the paper. Keeping this in mind, start by collating figure panels together based on their common message. In the main figures, show only what is essential to support the central finding of the figure; extraneous information will cloud the main message and frustrate the impatient reader.

Over the course of my PhD, one thing that has consistently surprised me is the importance of figure aesthetics. It does not matter how compelling the data is if the representation is unclear or crowded. Invest time in trying different representations of the data (e.g., replace the barplot with a dot matrix or heatmap) and design schemas to make it easier to understand the experiment or results. Running different representations by colleagues that are not closely involved with the project is a good way to find out which data representation works best to convey the intended message.

Similarly, articulating the rationale for your experimental plan can seem unnecessary when it is in fact essential to ensuring your reader's comprehension. One piece of advice is to select a few papers that you enjoyed reading because of the authors' clarity and writing style, and then attempt to emulate this structure or narrative style. Another is to play a game of *Jeopardy!*: while writing, derive a question for each of the statements you make. If the questions seem inadequate or unrelated to your central research question, this may suggest that you need to revise your statements.

Another helpful resource is to read reviewer comments for papers submitted by other members of your lab or by close collaborators. Reading reviewer comments can provide useful insights and help you to improve your experiments, analyses, and paper structure and style before submission, particularly for projects that share similar research techniques, methodologies, or analyses to your own project.

5. Avert interpersonal conflicts

Science today is a collaborative endeavor. Having worked on papers with many coauthors, I know that a big part of doing good science is being able to work effectively with different individuals. And sometimes, interpersonal conflicts can be the hardest part about getting a paper to the finish line. I don't pretend to have all the answers, but I do want to share a few observations about what made working together more productive and enjoyable.

Set clear expectations and boundaries from the beginning, including discussing authorship with your supervisor at the start of the project and throughout the paper's development. Remember too that although it's important to work collaboratively, it's also important for individual contributions to be recognized. Delineating separate tasks can make everyone feel that their contribution is of consequence, particularly when there is an overlap in expertise. Similarly, try to ensure that the team is on the same page and that everyone feels included in achieving the overall project aims.

Try to be open-minded and to not take critiques personally. Remind yourself occasionally that the people critiquing your data representation or interpretation are on *your* team. They want this project and paper to succeed like you do. If, after you have seriously and soberly considered their feedback, you still disagree, then make the effort of explaining your reasoning. Even if they continue to disagree, they will respect your efforts to persuade them, and your personal relationship won't be as affected by the discussion.

Get to know the working styles of your colleagues and supervisor(s). Everyone has a slightly different way of working: some are detail-oriented, some work better at night, some like updates regularly, some prefer to discuss data in person, etc. While it's impossible to accommodate everybody's preferences, going the extra mile will often yield a more productive interaction. What is universally true is that nobody fares well in long meetings without breaks or replenishment!

Be helpful when you can, without expecting anything in return. It's easy to become overwhelmed with your own projects, particularly as MD-PhD students with defined graduate timelines. It can be difficult to pull yourself away to help a colleague troubleshoot their experiment or review their manuscript. However, it's important to do so as a member of the research community. Also, you never know what benefits that interaction might bring in the future.

6. Use feedback constructively

The finishing touches precede the submission stage and can be nerve-wracking. Consider the comments provided by coauthors, particularly recurrent comments, but don't get overwhelmed or drawn in too many directions. Your supervisor will play an important role setting a direction for the revisions needed before submission. It is also important to practice the saying, "Don't let the perfect be the enemy of the good." There are always additional experiments that can be performed to strengthen the paper, but this needs to be balanced with a consideration for the essential evidence that supports the paper's conclusions and an appropriate timeline for the paper's publication.

7. Peer review: I can see the light!

Renovating the house after receiving reviewer and editor comments can be disruptive but should ultimately lead to a stronger and better supported publication. Be open-minded to reviewer comments. If they misunderstood a key aspect of your paper, consider the possibility that the relevant figure or text may need to be revised for clarity. Be polite and clear when addressing reviewer comments, acknowledging their expertise, explaining results from new experiments and analyses, and justifying why you believe some experiments or analyses are outside the scope of your paper.

Rejections by editors and reviewers are a natural part of the process. While you and your colleagues and supervisor will undoubtedly celebrate the publication of your paper, remember to celebrate the smaller milestones throughout the process. There are many lows in research, and it is equally important to celebrate the smaller breakthroughs with your team to motivate everyone to get to the finish line. Hopefully at the end of this process, you will be the proud parent of a scientific paper nurtured from conception to maturity.

CONCLUSION

You will probably have unfinished and ongoing projects at the conclusion of your PhD. Before transitioning back to medical school, ensure that you have the necessary support from your supervisor, fellow lab members, and collaborators to be able to complete these projects and publish during medical school. Prepare early for this transition, which is further discussed in Chapter 18, by providing the necessary project information and training to your team members.

Lastly, although this chapter focused on the importance of publishing well during graduate school, remember that your scientific worth is not solely defined by your publication record. There are many factors beyond a student's control when it comes to successfully publishing papers. The skill set acquired during a PhD should serve you well in the future, regardless of your graduate publication record.

14

Maintaining Clinical Knowledge, Skills, and Understanding During the PhD Training Years

Ethan Cottrill • Olive Tang

Ethan Cottrill *is a fifth-year MD-PhD student at Johns Hopkins University. His PhD research is in biomedical engineering and centers on developing new bone graft substitute materials. Prior to medical school, Ethan completed a bachelor of science in chemistry from Ohio University and a master of science in education from Johns Hopkins University.*

Olive Tang *is a fifth-year MD-PhD student at Johns Hopkins Bloomberg School of Public Health. Her PhD research is in cardiovascular epidemiology with a focus on the use of biomarkers in risk stratification. Prior to medical school, Olive completed a bachelor of arts in molecular and cellular biology from Harvard University.*

WHAT YOU NEED TO KNOW

- During your PhD training, actively seeking out opportunities to maintain your clinical skills is the best way to stay sharp and be ready for the transition back to medical school.

- Keep in touch with the clinical world to stay aware of your unique position as a future physician-scientist, a bridge between the worlds of research and the bedside.

- Clinical enrichment opportunities that you can do on your own include: reviewing the most high yield of your preclinical notes/resources, practicing your physical exam and interviewing skills, reading high-impact medical journals, and subscribing to medical news feeds.

- Clinical enrichment opportunities that are available at your medical institution include: shadowing attending physicians; participating in elective clerkships; attending departmental grand rounds; engaging with your medical school's student interest groups; participating in clinical research opportunities; and attending medical school/resident lectures, workshops, and skills-building sessions.

- Clinical enrichment opportunities that are available outside of your medical institution include: attending professional conferences and professional society meetings.

INTRODUCTION

For most students in an MD-PhD training program, the PhD training is sandwiched between MD training years. Despite this, the PhD training can feel relatively isolated from any clinical exposure. It is often a concern among students that they will become rusty on the clinical knowledge and skills acquired during the preclinical years of medical school. These include physical exam skills, interviewing techniques, and general medical knowledge outside the student's specific graduate area of research. As the first years of medical school grow more distant with progression of the PhD, a student's medical acumen may decline, making the transition back to medical school (a topic of Chapters 18–22) somewhat challenging and daunting. This chapter focuses on ways to maintain—or even enhance—clinical knowledge, skills, and understandings during the graduate school years.

This chapter is broken up into three categories. These are opportunities that (1) can be done relatively independently, (2) are likely available at one's medical institution, and (3) are available outside of one's medical institution. Our list is not exhaustive, and these opportunities may vary depending on the medical institution and training environment. That said, we hope that this can serve as a guiding framework.

CLINICAL ENRICHMENT OPPORTUNITIES THAT YOU CAN DO ON YOUR OWN

In this section, we describe opportunities for maintaining clinical acumen during graduate school that can be done relatively independently, from just about anywhere, using the resources you may already have available. These include: reviewing the most high yield of your preclinical notes/resources, practicing your physical exam and interviewing skills, reading high-impact medical journals, and subscribing to medical news feeds.

If you are anything like us, you probably will not be revisiting every single little note you ever jotted down during medical school (even though, for some reason, you are still hesitant to part with them). However, there are many high-yield ways you can review to maintain your clinical acumen.

Staying sharp

The first of these is *First Aid for the USMLE Step 1* and similar study guides, which focus on high-yield points that have been distilled down for the United States Medical Licensing Exam (USMLE) Step 1. Reviewing this book again during the PhD years is an excellent, self-guided way to stay sharp on the foundations of medicine. For example, committing to reading even one chapter per month over the course of a PhD can substantially reinforce a student's understanding of medical concepts. Other resources include question banks and flashcards used while studying for Step 1, such as free online resources like Anki. The field of online resources is rapidly expanding, with new companies entering the field at rapid rates. Indeed, many Step 1 study resources available today are offered as online and/or mobile applications; having such a resource on your mobile device provides a convenient way to review medical concepts at just about any time and in any place—for example, while waiting for that one experiment to finish!

In addition, for most students in an MD-PhD training program, the preclinical years are not restricted to book work on the scientific foundations of medicine. Students also learn interviewing and physical exam skills in preparation for the clinical years. Staying competent on these skills can be done at the lab or home with friends and family. Many "History of Present Illness" and "Physical Exam" templates/checklists are available online, if not provided by your medical school. Like reviewing key medical concepts, practicing these physical exam maneuvers or role-playing medical scenarios with friends and/or family members even once a month can help to maintain your clinical skills.

Staying up-to-date

Another relatively independent way to maintain—or even enhance—clinical acumen during the PhD years is by reading articles, or at least the abstracts, from high-impact medical journals. PhD students arguably should be reading these anyway, especially in their areas of research. Many articles published in these journals change the practice of medicine. Keeping abreast of recent medical advances in diverse fields can be extremely helpful and in general is a good habit to develop. In some cases, significant shifts in medicine may occur over the course of one's PhD, and staying informed of these changes can not only enhance one's understanding of medicine, but also ease the transition back to medical school. Furthermore, many of these journals pose regular questions in the form of case presentations to the readership (e.g., *The New England Journal of Medicine*'s "Question of the Week" and *JAMA: The Journal of the American Medical Association*'s "Clinical Challenge"), which often highlight the most recent guidelines in medical practice. Engaging with these questions is an excellent way to enhance clinical acumen, regardless of one's stage of training.

Don't forget about the ongoing medical research at your own institution. Most institutions will have highlights published in print or electronically (e.g., weekly email communication). Knowing what medical advances are being made at your institution not only broadens your medical exposure but also potentially offers an opportunity to find and establish research collaborations, which may accelerate your own medical discoveries.

Lastly, many news feeds (e.g., EurekAlert! and Newswise) are dedicated to promoting recent, important medical discoveries. Exploring these resources in a self-guided manner may not only enhance medical acumen, but also spark potential new research ideas during the PhD years.

CLINICAL ENRICHMENT OPPORTUNITIES AT YOUR MEDICAL INSTITUTION

Generally speaking, clinical enrichment opportunities likely abound at your medical institution, which, for most MD-PhD students, includes the medical school and one or more associated teaching hospitals. It is important to remember that, even during the PhD years, an MD-PhD student is still a medical student, albeit one on a somewhat lengthy leave of absence. Most MD-PhD students still get to keep their white coats and maintain access to the medical school and parts of the hospital.

Some MD-PhD students may have a sense, if not complete certainty, of their potential clinical interests by the start of the PhD or shortly thereafter. They may be conducting research in that area and have begun to steer their clinical and research training in the general direction they wish to go. Many clinical departments look fondly upon MD-PhD students who are interested in their specialty and are welcoming of them during their PhD years. Thus, a variety of clinical enrichment opportunities may be available including: shadowing attending physicians; participating in elective clerkships; attending departmental grand rounds; engaging with your medical school's student interest groups; participating in clinical research opportunities; and attending medical school/resident lectures, workshops, and skills-building sessions.

For those who have decided on their medical specialty or general field of interest, it may be easier to decide which clinical enrichment opportunities to pursue. For example, if a student is interested in surgery, shadowing a surgeon and engaging in surgical skills workshops may be particularly worthwhile and enjoyable experiences, and may motivate the student's pursuit of research efforts. However, during the graduate training phase, many MD-PhD students may not have decided what medical specialty they wish to pursue, or whether they wish to pursue a residency at all. If you are one these students, the PhD years may offer substantial value in affording you the time to engage in diverse clinical experiences across a broad range of medical specialties to further explore and define potential areas of clinical interest.

Shadowing

Shadowing an attending physician at your medical institution is one of the most effective ways to gain direct clinical exposure during the PhD years and may be done during rounds, in the clinic, and/or in the operating room. Shadowing generally involves asking an attending physician for permission to join their team for a morning, a day, or even weeks at a time. Furthermore, depending on your relationship with the attending physician and the setting, you may be allowed or encouraged to conduct the interview and physical exam and present the findings to the attending physician, similar to the clinical years of medical school. If you have completed a clinical clerkship prior to starting your graduate years, it may be easier to actively engage in the clinical care of the patients (with permission from the team, of course). For students interested in surgery, it may be possible to scrub into a surgical case with an attending surgeon, though this should be confirmed with one's MD-PhD training program.

In our experiences, shadowing can be particularly valuable to help refocus your attention on patient care. Improving patient care is the ultimate goal of much of our research, and a gentle reminder of that can be helpful during the PhD. Clinical exposure may be most beneficial when set up as an ongoing experience with the same mentor to minimize time spent reaching out to other mentors, organizing opportunities, and adjusting to the structure of different teams. If you have a practicing physician for a PhD thesis advisor, it may be easier to arrange to shadow your own research mentor in the clinic and gain valuable, first-hand experience with the important role of the physician-scientist in the hospital or in clinic during the PhD years.

Elective clerkship

In addition, some MD-PhD programs have formal elective, longitudinal clerkships that can be taken during the PhD years to involve students in regular (e.g., weekly) clinical experiences. For example, the Johns Hopkins School of Medicine offers a Lewisohn Longitudinal Elective in Continuity of Care, in which students work with a clinician for one half-day in the clinic every week over the course of a year. This experience is specifically designed for medical students pursuing one or more years of research training during medical school and essentially functions as a medical apprenticeship during the research years.

Formalized clerkships such as these can help facilitate more longitudinal relationships with a medical team and allow students to become more actively integrated into a clinical setting. Furthermore, just as research is inevitably more productive when there is protected time allocated to it, having dedicated time set aside for clinical training can be beneficial. An additional and simple way to maintain/enhance clinical acumen during the PhD years is to attend departmental (e.g., medical) ground rounds, which often meet weekly in the hospital. These meetings often include presentations by medical students (e.g., subinterns), residents, and attending physicians on patients with unique medical histories and/or recent advances in the field. They are, in our opinion, certainly high yield regardless of one's stage in MD-PhD training.

Staying involved

Other opportunities to integrate clinical experiences during the PhD years include staying (or becoming) involved in student interest groups (e.g., surgery interest group or internal medicine interest groups) at your medical school. These groups often organize fun, educational activities for all years of medical students, including hosting distinguished speakers (e.g., the department chairperson), coordinating match panels with graduating medical students, and conducting workshop and skills sessions (e.g., suture skills workshops). From our experience, first- and second-year medical students are particularly welcoming of MD-PhD students in these settings, as the MD-PhD students are often able to share helpful advice concerning research and to help maintain the institutional memory for these interest groups (by virtue of having a longer training trajectory) .

For MD-PhD students who wish to learn clinical research skills during the course of their training, engaging in clinical research projects (e.g., retrospective/prospective cohort studies) could be opportune and complement their thesis work. For example, an MD-PhD student conducting basic biomedical science research on new bone graft materials for spinal fusion may also want to perform clinical research studies investigating risk factors for failed fusion. These projects often provide excellent opportunities for students to integrate clinical experiences into their graduate training in a way that enhances their knowledge and understanding about a particular area of medicine.

Lastly, interested MD-PhD students may be able to attend resident or physician-scientist training program lectures, workshops, and skill sessions after requesting such access. These experiences may provide outstanding clinical exposure during the PhD years, offer contact with physician-scientists further ahead in training, and reinforce your desire for a particular career trajectory.

CLINICAL ENRICHMENT OPPORTUNITIES THAT ARE AVAILABLE OUTSIDE OF YOUR MEDICAL INSTITUTION

There are also a number of valuable opportunities available beyond the walls of your institution. After all, an MD-PhD training is a stepping stone on your professional journey. As you delve into your graduate studies, you will undoubtedly have opportunities to attend conferences hosted by various professional societies. These are wonderful opportunities to not only meet your fellow researchers, but also interface with practicing clinicians. Not all conferences will have a clinical focus, but many of the large professional societies, including the American Heart Association, American Diabetes Association, American Association of Neurological Surgeons, and Canadian Medical Association, just to name a few, have conferences that are well attended and intended for clinicians as well as researchers. These are often excellent arenas to witness the intricate interweaving of clinical medicine and investigative research. With the support of your research mentor, seek opportunities to attend and present at these conferences.

Furthermore, other professional societies, including the American College of Physicians and American College of Surgeons, also host events targeted at medical students and resident trainees. Often, there are meet-and-greets with residents, fellows, and attending physicians, social events that span multiple institutions, and practical clinical sessions or poster contests for trainees. These events often present excellent opportunities to build professional networks with scientific and clinical mentors.

CONCLUSION

In summary, there are numerous opportunities to integrate clinical experiences into an MD-PhD student's graduate training years. We encourage students to seek out these activities while ensuring the timely completion of the PhD training. We believe such experiences can bring great joy and meaning to an already intensely fulfilling stage of training and life. Good luck!

15

Completing Your Project

Stephanie Totten • Jiameng Xu

Stephanie Totten *is in the sixth year of the MD-PhD program at McGill University. Her doctoral research is in the field of breast cancer metabolism and focuses on exploring and characterizing rational combination therapies that sensitize tumors to the metabolic drug phenformin. Prior to starting the double program, Stephanie completed her bachelor's degree in life sciences and her master's degree in experimental medicine at McGill University.*

Jiameng Xu *is in the seventh year of the MD-PhD program at McGill University. She has recently completed her PhD dissertation, an ethnographic study based in an inpatient psychiatry unit, which captures the lived experience of persons living with mental illness and their family members. She has also been involved in initiatives to create a space for the arts and humanities within health professional training and in spaces of health care delivery.*

INTRODUCTION

This chapter is organized in a question-and-answer style and was written as a collaboration between Stephanie Totten and Jiameng Xu. As we decided how to integrate our sections together over coffee one evening, it became apparent that in spite of differences in the topics and methodologies of our PhDs, there were many common themes. We both agreed on how

---

WHAT YOU NEED TO KNOW

- Ask for advice prior to starting and throughout your PhD.
- Start early. If possible, start part time in the lab before dedicated research time begins and apply for scholarships early. If you are doing field-based research, prioritize establishing contact with your field site early in your PhD.
- Test out your data as you go. Make figures, keep track of references and methods, and write early and often.
- Develop your own strategies for staying on track. Set goals. Think long-term (yearly) and short-term (daily). Goals related to achieving your project aims, as well as related to your overall development as a doctoral student (coursework, workshops, conferences, soft-skill development).
- Make wellness a priority. Take breaks and vacation, exercise, sleep, eat well, and maintain interests and relationships outside of your research and lab. You will be a better researcher for it!

useful it has been to ask for advice and input from mentors and colleagues before and during our degrees.

The strategies outlined in this chapter regarding completing your project are a combination of the advice we have individually received from mentors, colleagues, and senior graduate students, as well as some of the lessons we have learned through our experience thus far. We present suggestions specific to conducting a PhD in two different disciplines and their differing modalities, with Stephanie writing from her work in the wet lab in cancer biology, and Jiameng writing from her PhD involving ethnographic fieldwork. While the suggestions herein do not encompass all possible methodologies and PhD paths that MD-PhD students may take, we aim to highlight the differences between our two respective methodologies. We hope the reader can extrapolate from these suggestions for their work in their own fields. Additionally, we hope these questions can guide you in potential discussions with colleagues and mentors as you prepare for the exciting journey that is your PhD.

As you read through this chapter, there are several common general suggestions we agreed upon during our discussion, the details of which are outlined below, although we provide our unique perspectives, informed by our PhD experiences. Furthermore, we agreed whole-heartedly that maintaining wellness throughout our PhD training was most fundamental to our doctoral research experiences, addressed at the chapter's end. Advice is simply a sugges-tion, and a single suggestion will not apply to all situations or to all individuals. Our hope is that after reading this chapter, you will feel empowered to ask for advice, integrate the suggestions in a way that works for you, and take ownership and make the most of your PhD.

WHAT ARE YOUR RESEARCH EXPERIENCES TO DATE?

Stephanie

At the time of writing this chapter, I am completing the fourth year of my PhD under the supervision of Josie Ursini-Siegel, PhD, at the Lady Davis Institute at the Jewish General Hospital (I am a sixth-year student in the combined MD-PhD program). Early clinical expe-riences as an MD-PhD student in the breast clinic confirmed my desire to dedicate myself to addressing some of the key knowledge gaps in breast cancer treatment resistance, metastasis, and tumor metabolism. Dr. Ursini-Siegel's lab was a natural fit. She is a dedicated mentor, with a productive, well-funded, and collaborative lab. My colleagues, who soon became good friends, were extremely supportive. Prior to enrolling in the combined program under the supervision of Natalie Johnson, MD, PhD, and performed undergraduate summer research and a senior undergraduate research project under the supervision of Armando Jardim, PhD, at McGill's Institute of Parasitology.

Jiameng

During my undergraduate studies in life sciences at Queen's University, I chose a spe-cialization in neuroscience during the third and fourth years. Under the supervision of Dr. Georg Northoff at the University of Ottawa, I conducted research using functional magnetic resonance imaging with human research participants. I also conducted research into the mechanism of central sensitization of inflammatory pain in inflammatory bowel disease, using mouse models, with Dr. Alan Lomax at Queen's University. At the time, I wanted to gain training in multiple modalities of investigation. I was interested in inves-tigating empirically subjectivity and experience. During the first year of medical school, when I was trying to figure out where I wanted to do my PhD, I realized that I needed to learn how to understand experience in a radically different way from how I was taught—that is, via quantitative and experimental methods. This desire led me to work with my PhD advisor, Dr. Melissa Park, and to throw myself into the world of ethnography and methods of inquiring into experience by sharing such experiences with the people in my study.

HOW CAN YOU GET HELPFUL ADVICE?

Stephanie

Don't be shy ask seniors in the program, students who've graduated, lab members, and even established professors what their suggestions are regarding graduate school and what worked for them. I love getting different perspectives and integrating what I have heard. Some advice will work for you, some won't, and some you won't even try. However, it is my experience that speaking with different people who have gone through the same or similar training as you provides invaluable insight to help guide you. In fact, most of the advice and suggestions within this chapter resulted from asking many people for their advice!

Jiameng: I have received helpful advice by voicing my anxiety about an aspect of my project

For example, My thesis advisor gave me this advice sometime during the first six months of my PhD program. We were sitting at a table in her office, looking over a yearly tracking progress form that we had to submit to the department. I was worried about the time pressure and that I would not be able to complete the work I felt I needed to do. I must have been trying to fit too many ideas together, when Melissa said with a smile, "Your PhD will follow you for the rest of your life, but treat it as an appetizer. I know you will continue thinking about these questions." Hearing this, especially at the start of my PhD journey, deflated my anxiety. Thereafter, whenever I felt at risk of becoming paralyzed by the pressure I put on myself, I would repeat her advice and remember that the PhD is only the beginning of things. Focus on the process of inquiry, enjoy the ride. My task during the PhD was not to construct a monument, but to get a start, and to prepare for the exciting work that is yet to come. Voicing specific anxieties can be the best way to receive advice that can help you become unstuck.

WHY AND HOW SHOULD A STUDENT GET AN EARLY START ON THE TIME-INTENSIVE STAGES OF RESEARCH?

Stephanie

McGill's MD-PhD program allows for a maximum of 4 years of dedicated research time for the PhD component of the program. Considering this, my suggestion to make the most of your protected time is to start your project early. Once I had determined the lab and project I wanted to work on, I took advantage of time during preclinical medical school to start working in the lab. Several of my colleagues in the MD-PhD program at McGill did the same. Chapter 8 ("Starting Medical School and Integrating Research") contains some more advice on how you can balance early research with preclinical medical school. It has been my experience that getting used to a new lab environment and project can take some time.

If you're starting in a lab early, discuss this learning curve with your new supervisor, and ask about the possibilities of being paired with a senior graduate student or postdoc in the laboratory to be trained. My supervisor Josie's lab is extremely collegial, and I was fortunate to be surrounded and trained by very kind and collaborative graduate students who later became dear friends.

I am grateful I chose to start in the lab early. My supervisor's research program relies heavily on transgenic mouse models to study breast cancer progression and tumor-stromal interactions. This method can take several months, with a lot of waiting time between the mouse breedings. Starting early and part-time in the lab was particularly beneficial for my situation. Maintaining a mouse colony and producing experimental mouse models, in my case, did not require long hours every day. Yet, through working part-time in the lab during medical school, I generated the mice necessary to address an important aspect of one of my projects and several experimental questions. In addition, I learned about the functioning of the lab and became familiar with some of the experimental techniques relevant to my project and ultimately, my training. I also had the great opportunity to assist a senior graduate student with some experiments for her publication, which afforded me authorship on a paper.

Ultimately, I feel that starting this work early saved me about a year of time during my PhD, and that when I officially started the PhD portion of my program, I felt more prepared to make the most of my protected research time. I recognize that not all projects are the same, and in the end my recommendation will always be to do what feels best for you. With that in mind, I firmly believe that any work you do to familiarize yourself with your project, lab, supervisor, or colleagues prior to starting your dedicated research time will be useful for you. Additionally, starting your research early is a good opportunity to confirm your choice of lab and supervisor. As addressed in Chapter 10, it is pivotal that the project, supervisor, and research team are compatible with your goals and expectations.

I also addressed potential hurdles to starting research during medical school. MD-PhD programs across North America vary in their sequencing of the required curriculum components for each degree. Here at McGill, medical school coursework is during the first one and a half years, with a schedule that allows for quite a lot of flexibility and independent study. Furthermore, the graduate student in Josie's lab who graciously agreed to train me would spend very long hours working at the lab, and therefore was almost always available to help me with any questions I had, even when my schedule only permitted me to be at the lab during late afternoon, evenings, and weekends. One potential limitation could be that current graduate students, research associates/assistants, or postdoctoral students in the lab who are responsible for training or supervising you may not be available during the times you are considering coming to the lab. This largely depends on how flexible your medical school schedule is and also the structure of the MD-PhD program at your school.

Alternative strategies exist. If starting benchwork during the first year of medical school is not possible or simply something that you decide is not right for you, then starting work during the summers prior to beginning the PhD portion of your degree is a really good alternative. Additionally, regardless of whether you commence benchwork prior to your dedicated research years or not, identifying your thesis topic early can be very helpful. Read Chapter 11 ("Defining Your Project") for more information on how to begin narrowing it down. The beginning of medical school can be an excellent time to start reading the relevant literature for your project and to apply for scholarships early! Research scholarship applications tend to take time to put together. Starting these early can also free up time for dedicated research in the future.

Jiameng

Conducting field-based research within a fixed time frame requires advanced planning. Field-based research is conducted in the actual contexts where organisms, including humans, live. It generates rich data and insights, but it can also be logistically challenging to carry out. At the beginning of my PhD, I was wondering if and how an ethnographic study—one type of field-based research—could be possible within the time frame of 4 years. Gaining entry into a field, establishing relationships, obtaining research ethics board approval, navigating ethical issues, grappling with emergent phenomena, and carrying out data collection and analysis concurrently are a small selection of the issues that field researchers face. In the suggestions below, I echo several of Stephanie's suggestions above, applying them here to field-based research.

It was also important to prioritize establishing contact with the field site early on in my study. In all domains of research, obtaining research ethics and proposal approval are milestones and take significant time, requiring multiple cycles of submissions and revisions. In field-based research, the particularities of the field site will directly influence the data collection methods and even the kinds of phenomena that can be studied. These particularities often cannot be adequately predicted until one enters the field site for the first time. For example, the discovery that you can no longer be stationed with a particular group of people due to external forces such as political conflict, or that your initial research question must be discarded because they do not capture what people are actually living, are distinct possibilities that field researchers may be confronted with at the outset of entering the field. Entering the field early can help you to gain essential contextual knowledge for designing your study. If possible, entering the field can occur in parallel with the earliest stages of the PhD, such as reviewing literature or completing required coursework.

There are many approaches to establishing contact with a field site. For some, it is to volunteer. For others, it is to request permission to be a visitor or observer. Each method carries with it an ethical duty to the people in the field. In my case, my PhD advisor brought me on as an "apprentice" in ongoing research activities that gave me early exposure to the field, allowing me to follow events, people, and the culture of what would eventually become my study field site. Entering the field as one of the first steps I took during the PhD allowed me to collect more in-depth data, because the people in the field were already familiar with me, and I had already formed a preliminary, working understanding of what is significant to them.

HOW CAN YOU ORGANIZE AND TEST OUT YOUR DATA AS YOUR RESEARCH PROGRESSES?

Stephanie: Make publishable figures and write methods as you generate data

In addition to keeping details of what you did, using separate word documents to write detailed methods in manuscript format can save you a lot of time when you write a manuscript or your thesis. Building figures has many advantages. For students doing their PhD in the basic sciences in particular, I found that combining your independent experimental replicates into a publishable graphing file (for example in GraphPad) as you generate the data can help save time when it comes to presentations, lab meetings, poster preparation, manuscripts, and tracking your work.

One strategy I adopted from a mentor and friend in the lab was to keep track of experimental repeats by having a folder with the question we were addressing, then subfolders with the experiment names. Within each of those were subfolders for pilots and n1, n2, n3, n4, etc. Within each of those, subfolders were created for pilot, and each biological repeat of the experiment (labeled n1, n2, n3, n4 etc). I include all files with methods, raw data and statistical analyses in the corresponding numbered biological repeat folder. Finally, once all biological repeats of that experiment are complete, I generate another additional folder for the combined analysis and corresponding Graphpad file. Taking the time to progressively group figures into figure panels as if you were writing a manuscript early on in your project, including anything you may consider supplemental data, can really aid in tracking your progress and guiding your future research. The order of things will most probably change, some data will be shuffled around to different sections, but in my experience, doing so may allow you to identify unanswered questions and priorities, and furthermore, is a great way to monitor of your progress throughout your basic science PhD. Additionally, keeping track of references and articles as you read the literature, for example, by using a reference software, like EndNote or Papers (addressed in Chapter 16), will save you a lot of time when you need to prepare presentations, write manuscripts, and compose your thesis. This collection of data can be useful from the very earliest moment you begin defining your project, as discussed in Chapter 11.

Jiameng: Develop a process for writing early and often

This suggestion mirrors Stephanie's advice of making figures summarizing the data throughout one's nascent work. The written text in social sciences and humanities research is analogous to data figures in quantitative and experimental research. Crafting the final written text, even when aided by coding and categorizing software programs, is unpredictable and can take longer than initially anticipated. Taking some time to develop a method for making notes, writing reflections and preliminary interpretations, and turning drafts into finalized pieces can provide a scaffolding for writing the dissertation. Part of making such a scaffolding is balancing writing against other activities, such as setting enough time for writing field notes when one is immersed in fieldwork (this sometimes necessitates resisting the pull of returning to the field to simply collect more data). Devising a process for analysis, interpretation, and writing can also lead you to envision how requisite academic activities can support your progress in your thesis work. For example, my advisor encouraged me to use presentations at research conferences as an opportunity to test out an analysis based upon a significant portion of my data.

A piece of advice I gleaned was to write early and often as a means of working out ideas. The segments of writing that I made prior to and throughout my fieldwork became invaluable in the writing of my thesis, especially when I noticed that certain ideas, questions, and references to literature recurred and took on significance I could not have foreseen. I took these ideas to be the most important ones and organized my data analysis, interpretation, and discussion around them. Following the advice of other qualitative researchers, I saved all correspondence, emails, initial jottings, and any reflections, no matter how fragmented or preliminary. Many of these became part of my dissertation. While the final 10 months of my PhD candidacy were spent in writing my dissertation, looking back now I see that writing early and often had actually allowed me to develop it over a longer span of time.

WHAT SPECIFIC STRATEGIES CAN HELP YOU TO STAY ON TRACK AND ORGANIZED DURING YOUR PhD?

Stephanie: Expect that many experiments will yield negative data

This is the reality. As I came to understand, negative data is very important and just as informative as positive data. The sooner I realized this, the easier things were, and importantly, the less time I wasted. I came to realize that instead of being focused on the results of a certain experiment, my energy was better spent ensuring that I was setting up well-planned and appropriately controlled experiments, and that would allow me to answer our particular research question.

Set project and learning goals

PhD training is often less structured than medical school. I found that setting a framework for my 4 years, including project and learning goals, has helped me progress throughout my PhD thus far. Setting goals from the beginning in terms of experimental aims, committee meetings, presentations/conferences, paper revisions, and teaching experiences enabled me to stay on track during my PhD. Being specific and detailed in formulating my goals was important for me. I want to highlight that in addition to goals for experiments and coursework, setting goals for professional development and for communicating my research through presentations, conferences, and seminars was also important in my training. In my experience, integrating these into your PhD will enrich your training, help move your project along, and provide great opportunities for feedback.

I am of the view that the more specific a goal is, the more likely you are to achieve it. As an example of goal setting, prior to starting my PhD, I set the goal of completing all of the course requirements for the degree by the start of my third year. Goals can and should be revised and edited, so even if the experimental aims change (which is highly probable), or attending a particular conference does not work out, aiming to attend a certain conference yearly will help you keep on track or push you to find alternatives. Perhaps the best analogy for setting goals during the PhD is the process of defining and refining them when training for a marathon. Training for long-distance races requires foresight, long-term planning, and adaptation. Unexpected injuries, personal events, and just life can and most probably will interfere with your perfectly designed training schedule. Just as in a running schedule, a PhD training schedule requires the same flexibility and editing of goals. Finally, planning well in advance and setting a framework to follow has really helped me (and will help you too).

Plan your week

Along the same line as goal setting, defining daily, weekly, and even monthly priorities, and regularly reviewing and editing them has been my method of choice for staying organized throughout my PhD. If you already have an organization tool of choice, stick with it or try out something new, like paper and pen, a calendar app of your choice, or my favorite, Microsoft OneNote. Be realistic about daily goals. That's something I'm still working on myself. Goals are incredibly important, but carefully thought-out and consistent daily habits are fundamental in achieving your goals. I found that keeping a separate log of ideas that come up during meetings and presentations, or just while reading was also very helpful.

Schedule regular meetings with the supervisor and advisory committee

Many doctoral programs will require that students have a thesis advisory committee. Depending on the university and particular program, the makeup of the thesis advisory committee can differ in terms of the number of committee members, whether they are assigned or can be selected by the student and their supervisor, etc. Additionally, many graduate programs have mandatory yearly meeting schedules along with particular policies regarding when these meetings should be held and what documents are required. Be sure to understand your particular situation and to schedule these group meetings well in advance (four months is typically what I aimed for). It is my experience that schedules of busy professors fill up very quickly. These yearly advisory meetings have been incredibly helpful for me thus far. My committee members are experts in their respective fields and provided great suggestions in terms of experiments and collaborations, and unique perspectives on interesting avenues to pursue.

In addition to these required meetings, my supervisor had a very open-door policy, making regular updates with her much easier. Every supervisor and student will be different, but I found that by doing regular updates with my supervisor, I kept on track, was able to get her input on any problems that occurred, and get her feedback on experimental priorities. I have found that supervisors have the experience and knowledge to identify potential problems before they happen.

Practice wellness

Finally, and certainly equally importantly, take time away from the lab and your studies. I firmly believe that in order to contribute in the best way one can during their PhD and to learn the most, one must stay physically and mentally healthy. It is simple: you will be more productive and engaged when you are rested and refreshed. My advice is to not wait until you are burned out to take a break and to integrate life outside of research into your daily habits. Whether taking a staycation or traveling somewhere distant, it's better to take a week or two off than to run at 50% capacity for a long time.

My partner, family, and close friends have supported me tremendously in my training thus far. I have also learned that maintaining healthy habits is critical to being engaged in the lab, the hospital, and in my personal life. Personally, this means eating a mostly plant-based diet, regular exercise, sufficient sleep, and incorporating different forms of rest into my day, week, and year. I firmly believe that maintaining relationships, hobbies, and interests outside of your work will make you a more engaged researcher and medical trainee.

Jiameng: Identify people to whom you can turn to work through emergent issues in the field and data analysis

Field-based research is processual. Issues and phenomena emerge that cannot be foreseen or anticipated and that may become incorporated into the study itself. The emergent issues, especially if they concern the well-being of people in the field or the researcher, can also be time-sensitive. It is important to have others that you can turn to for working through discussion issues that arise. Being able to turn to one's advisor, supervisory committee, peers, and other identified researchers and colleagues will help issues be addressed in a timely manner. For example, my advisor arranged with me that we touch base every Monday at 11 AM during my fieldwork. I could decide to contact her via text message, email, or telephone to ask her questions or simply let her know that things were okay. On two occasions, I called her from the field to discuss an emergent ethical issue. My regular discussions with my advisor and supervisory committee members helped me to cultivate a sense of confidence and closeness with my data that facilitated the writing of my research findings.

Keep learning and allowing yourself to try things that interest you

During the PhD, I stayed motivated by maintaining a parallel engagement in other domains. Earlier, we spoke collectively about coping with the time pressure of a PhD program, but paradoxically, taking time to do other things can help you to remain engaged and develop a wider perspective. For me, this involved activities in the medical humanities, continuing to write poetry, and taking opportunities to teach. For many of my graduate classmates, the PhD years were a time for trying new things and being a part of many intersecting communities. I watched as my fellow graduate, MD-PhD, and medical school classmates grappled with uncertainty about the future. This included uncertainty about the direction and outcomes of our research work and graduate training, about what career paths we may have, and about how we could ensure that the work we are doing is worthwhile to ourselves and the communities we aim to serve. For many of us, and possibly for you, a response to an uncertain future was to find things in the here and now that gave us meaning. Some learned a winter sport or new language; others organized around social justice causes or health issues.

Take time to look after yourself and the people you love

The period during my comprehensive exams—which in my department is structured as students being given 12 weeks to research and write three long, original essays—took a toll on my health. At the time, I felt guilty at the thought of taking time away from researching and writing my essays to do the things I loved, from long-distance running to gym classes with a friend, to taking the time to cook and eat healthy meals, to spending time with family and friends. During the final year of my PhD, when things became very busy once more, I set a goal for myself to protect other important aspects of my life from being eroded by the pressures of research work. I believe doing so helped me to complete my PhD and to feel that I was true to myself in the process.

At the time I started my PhD, I was at a point in my life when I wanted to strengthen my relationship with my family and to get to know them for who they are. Making this a priority also helped the PhD years to feel significant and rewarding. It was a privilege to share the journey with family members and friends, which also helped me to not feel alone. Toward the end of the third year of my PhD, my grandfather's health deteriorated rapidly, and he became terminally ill. For a couple of weeks, I felt torn between my responsibilities to the people in my academic life and to my grandfather and my family. The understanding, wisdom, and humanity of my advisor helped me to accept taking a brief respite from my fieldwork to be with my dying grandfather. Looking back now, I am grateful for making this decision. I think it also helped me to feel afterward that I could return to my work with a sense of integrity, as I knew I had already helped to accompany my family during this difficult time.

During my PhD, I also sought help from counseling services at my university, and then, during the final year of my PhD and after my grandfather's death, from more regular sessions with a counselor at a center in the community that offered a sliding scale. I was at first very reluctant to seek help, but after hearing the stories of other classmates and mentors, both in the research and medical communities, about the challenges they faced and how they learned to reach out for the support they needed, I felt more empowered to do the same. Doing so has helped me weather the challenges of both completing a PhD and the inevitable, unanticipated ups and downs of life that occur simultaneously as one aims to complete a long-term project. Though other students may not be facing the specific circumstances I had, I wanted to share that I benefited greatly from seeking help to maintain my mental and emotional well-being.

CONCLUSION: WHAT IS THE MOST IMPORTANT LESSON YOU LEARNED DURING YOUR PhD?

Stephanie: Self-compassion

My PhD provided me numerous learning experiences both in and outside of research, some expected, others that came as complete and (mostly) welcome surprises. One such surprise was my discovery of Dr. Kristin Neff's work on self-compassion. I was resistant at first. As reluctant as I am to admit this now, when I first read the term "self-compassion," it seemed to lend itself as an excuse to be less productive, less hard-working and to not uphold responsibility in personal relationships. However, by trusting in the person that recommended it and working hard to open my mind and heart to Dr. Neff's book, *Self-Compassion: The Proven Power of Being Kind to Yourself*, I gained a completely new perspective. What I came to realize is that my inner-critic voice had occupied many of my thoughts and actions, and with a lot of practice, working to let that voice go actually allowed me to be more productive at work and more present in my personal life. Through practicing self-compassion, I came to experience compassion for others in a completely different way. I highly encourage you to read her book and explore the concept for yourself. The saying "we cannot give to others what we first do not give to ourselves" has become a motto that I often return to and a reminder to continue my self-compassion practice, not only for myself, but also for my loved ones, colleagues, and future patients.

Jiameng: That I am not alone

The last year of my PhD, when I was intensively writing a dissertation that would eventually number almost 80,000 words, was very challenging. During that time I carried an image in my mind that I thought would carry me through the process. During that last year, as I was striving to make some meaning from the data I had, I felt as though I was sailing on a boat surrounded by fog. As the months wore on, the fog gradually began to lift, and the image turned to one not of isolation, but having people standing on the shore who were waiting for me. These included my classmates and PhD advisor, the research participants, friends, and family. On the shore, as well, were the authors and other researchers, living and dead, who have had a hand in this work. On that shore were also people I have never met, living in another place and time, who might one day want to know that this work has been done. Although the PhD journey has given me much time alone to complete it, it ultimately helped me to learn how my work is part of a tradition of inquiry. Even as the PhD is a journey to become an independent scholar, it shows us how we are profoundly connected to others.

16

Thesis Writing

Anonymous

Anonymous is a fifth-year MD-PhD student at McGill University. Before beginning his dual-degree program, he completed an engineering degree. His research interests include medical imaging analysis and medical informatics. His research involves modeling the way the brain changes naturally over the life span.

INTRODUCTION

This chapter presents a brief overview of a doctoral thesis and provides useful tips and suggestions on the writing process. During thesis writing, the steps detailed in the past few chapters, particularly Chapter 11 ("Defining Your Project"), Chapter 12 ("Maximizing Research Productivity"), and Chapter 15 ("Completing Your Project") are integrated into a final product. MD-PhD students should read this chapter before beginning the PhD phase of the dual program, because the advice given here is more useful the earlier it is adopted.

THESIS COMMITTEE

The thesis supervisory committee exists to provide constructive criticism to the student throughout the PhD. Their importance was also addressed in Chapter 11, and for good reason; they should be enriching your project practically from start to finish. The full committee is composed of the student's thesis supervisor(s) and one or more additional faculty members. Students should choose committee members who have sufficient knowledge of the field to provide meaningful insight and advice; sufficient availability to attend annual progress tracking meetings and provide feedback on papers, the thesis proposal, and the thesis itself; and who do not possess a conflict of interest with the thesis supervisor(s) or the student.

WHAT YOU NEED TO KNOW

- Follow your school's specific guidelines for the structure of your thesis.
- Write early, write often.
- Choose a citation-management software.
- Keep your reference list up-to-date, starting from your initial literature review.
- Don't neglect yourself: make time for friends, family, and fun, and stay active.

Choosing committee members with complementary knowledge and background is a sound strategy. For example, having a clinician on the committee can help your thesis have a well-planned clinical applicability. A faculty member from the MD-PhD program should also serve on the thesis supervisory committee. Their job will be to ensure that the unique circumstances of the joint program are known to the committee members (such as the transition from full-time PhD studies to full-time clinical studies at the end of the third or fourth year of graduate studies).

In addition to providing constructive criticism and feedback on papers and the thesis, the committee also evaluates the academic progress of the student and helps to plan specific objectives during each committee meeting. The thesis committee is expected to meet as least once a year. Near the end of the PhD, the thesis committee will also review and approve the thesis.

For my committee, in addition to my two co-supervisors, I chose a clinician, a mentor from the MD-PhD program, and a domain expert. Having a large committee can make scheduling my committee meetings a challenge, but I believe the extra knowledge and advice that can be provided by this group is well worth the effort.

Thesis requirements

The requirements for a PhD thesis vary between departments and schools. This section will detail some of the common thesis requirements. The thesis for a doctoral degree must present original research that makes a distinct contribution to knowledge in the field, as well as demonstrate familiarity with the previous work in that field. The thesis must also be structured in a logical manner and clearly demonstrate the ability to plan and carry out original research, including the ability to present and defend the results and conclusions of the research. While there are not usually length requirements for PhD theses, they are expected to be as concise as possible, as concision is one expected aspect of doctoral research.

DIFFERENT THESIS STYLES

A thesis can be written in the traditional monograph style or in a manuscript-based style. In the traditional monograph style, the thesis is structured into specific chapters that each present an important aspect of the project. In a manuscript-based thesis, individual papers are included. For a manuscript-based thesis, each included paper should contribute an important aspect of the thesis. All the work should be discussed in a comprehensive discussion section without simply repeating the discussion from the manuscripts.

Your school or department may have specific requirements or standards for the number of included articles for a manuscript-based thesis. Additionally, your school likely has a requirement that the student is the sole first author on each included paper. For situations where the student is not the sole first author on a publication, the school will likely recommend that the student write a monograph-based thesis.

The decision to write either a traditional-style or manuscript-based thesis should be made early and in consultation with the student's supervisor(s) and thesis committee. A traditional monograph-style thesis allows a greater flexibility in the order of presentation of the materials and methods used. If a manuscript-based thesis is chosen, the publishable components of the project need to be identified early, and these components should be integrated into the design of the research project. Timelines for publication are important to note, as some schools may only allow published or submitted manuscripts to be included in a thesis.

As we naturally write manuscripts during our PhD studies, writing a manuscript-based thesis can save considerable time and effort. For this reason, I chose it for both my master's and PhD theses.

SAMPLE THESIS STRUCTURE AND COMPONENTS

While this section presents recommendations for the structure of a PhD thesis, make sure to follow your university's thesis guidelines. Be careful not to copy the structure and components of another thesis from your school, as thesis requirements can change over time. Always refer to the thesis requirements published by your university.

The following components must be present in a thesis:

- I. Title page
- II. Table of contents
- III. Abstract
- IV. Acknowledgments
- V. Contribution to original knowledge
- VI. Contribution of authors
- VII. Introduction
- VIII. Comprehensive literature review
- IX. Methodology
- X. Research findings
- XI. Discussion
- XII. Conclusion/summary
- XIII. Reference list

The title page of a thesis must state the title of the thesis. Additionally, the student's name, department/division/program, and university must be listed along with the month and year the thesis was submitted. Your school will also likely have a statement and copyright notice that are required for this page.

The table of contents should reference the major sections of your thesis, including the abstract, lay summary (if included), chapter or section headings, references, and appendices. A list of tables, figures, and illustrations should also be included and listed in the table of contents. If a list of symbols and abbreviations (or glossary) is included, it should be placed after the list of figures and tables and be included in the table of contents.

In the acknowledgments section, the student must declare any and all assistance that he or she received during the writing of the thesis, whether the assistance was paid for or not. The help may have come from fellow students, staff, research assistants, committee members, mentors, or collaborators. The assistance may have been for any phase of the thesis project: the collection of data or specimens, design of the experiment, conduction of the experiment, data analysis, or writing of the thesis or included manuscripts. In addition to these requirements, the advice and guidance provided by the thesis supervisor(s) and advisors should be acknowledged.

A doctoral thesis must demonstrate original scholarship and contribute to the knowledge of the field. The thesis should clearly state what aspects of it are considered original. The thesis must also clearly state the contributions made to each chapter and included manuscripts. In addition to detailing the contributions that the student made to each chapter and manuscript, the contributions by any coauthors must also be explicitly stated.

The objective and rationale behind the project should be clearly and succinctly stated in the introduction to the thesis. A comprehensive review of the literature of the field should be provided as well. Whether a monograph-style or manuscript-based thesis is being written, the main body of the thesis should clearly state the methods used and the specific and noteworthy findings. Following the sections denoting the methods and results, a comprehensive discussion section must be written that places the results in the context of the field. A concise conclusion details the implications of the findings and summarizes the main points of the research and how each specific objective was met.

THESIS WRITING TIPS

Many students hate writing. If, like me, you are one of these people, my first tip to you is to develop a writing plan at the beginning of your thesis. In addition to creating a plan for your entire thesis, having specific goals for each semester will help you stay on target. Breaking down these goals into weekly or monthly plans with manageable and specific tasks should help prevent you from falling behind. In addition to developing a writing plan, many students find it beneficial to develop the habit of writing every day. Even if you just write a few sentences, developing this habit can help change your thinking and help you better understand your thought process by forcing you to put your thoughts down in a coherent fashion.

Another useful tip is to make sure you write as you go. In other words, make sure you progress toward each of the main parts of your thesis as you progress through your project. At the beginning of your project, as addressed in Chapter 11, perform your initial literature search, organize it in your favorite citation-management software (see the following section for recommendations), and write an initial literature review. As you continue to read more and more literature, continue adding new sections and specific details to your literature review. You will find it an invaluable resource as a place to review your knowledge. Similarly, while you are conducting experiments, carefully document your methodology. This will be useful not just for your thesis but also for writing those articles which we are required to publish or perish!

Organize your thoughts as they occur to you in a place that is easy to access. Some options for organization include Google Keep as an app on your smartphone, the iOS Notes app, the Trello project-management app, Microsoft OneNote, or an old school-paper notebook. The place where you store your notes is not what matters; what matters is that you make sure you don't lose track of any sudden inspirations or thoughts that occur to you. You never know when a new idea might inspire a new experiment or help you resolve a quandary that you've been pondering for a considerable amount of time.

Start using a citation-management software from the very first day of your PhD project. It might seem like an inconvenience, but it will save you an incredible amount of time when you are actively writing. Also consider writing short abstracts in your own words for each article you read. Writing even a short two-sentence description of what you consider the most important aspects of the work will allow you to quickly review an incredible amount of pertinent information.

Don't assume you're an expert in writing. Your university likely offers workshops on writing tailored specifically to graduate students. The writing center at your university should also offer consultations with experienced writers for help in editing your work. In addition to these resources provided by your school, you can find an almost unlimited supply of advice online by searching for terms such as "thesis writing suggestions," "how-to guide for scientific writing," etc. The more you read about how to write, the more ideas and strategies you'll have at your disposal.

Writing anything is a process of writing and revising. While you may write sections at the beginning of your project that eventually become irrelevant as your research focus is revised, this is part of the revision process, and having more to work with is better than having nothing. Take note of exemplary writing as you read the literature of your field and write down what struck you as noteworthy. As you attend courses on writing and collaborate with fellow researchers, make an effort to find others who can reliably edit your drafts. The more people who review your work, the more constructive criticism you will receive and the better your final draft will be. Senior students, lab staff, and your PhD supervisor and committee members are excellent sources for guidance and to ask to read your drafts and provide writing advice.

After writing a significant length of text, make sure to take a break before coming back to revise it. A fresh, well-rested mind will notice errors much more reliably than a fatigued one. Also, because a thesis takes a long time to read, you should submit sections of your thesis to your supervisor to read and edit. This will help you avoid worrying about submission deadlines near the end of your thesis preparation.

Do not have any zero days (days where no progress is made) during your PhD (this applies to every phase of your PhD, not just when writing). If you are too tired to write, double-check your references. Even the smallest task is important. Just putting in a few minutes' worth of work to do a minor task (such as adding a caption to a figure) may overcome your mental hurdles and help shift you into productive gear.

This tip is the most important of all: Make sure that you look after yourself during this stressful and anxiety-ridden process. The news and literature are full of evidence of the stress experienced by graduate students. Make sure you are proactive in combating it by eating well, exercising frequently, and engaging in your hobbies. Also, remember to go outside for fresh air and sunlight.

CITATION-MANAGEMENT SOFTWARE

This section details different citation managers that are available to help you organize your reference library while writing your thesis. The major software citation managers highlighted in this section are EndNote, Mendeley, PaperPile, and Papers. The software to use depends on the software you will be using to write your manuscripts and thesis, as well as the operating system you will be writing on. The software options presented here are examples of popular software available for each major operating system, but the list is far from exhaustive. Consult with your university's librarians, as well as students and staff in your lab to learn what software is commonly used among your peers, as sharing citation-management software can make research and writing collaborations work more efficiently. The choice of software is also deeply personal, and I recommend students perform their own research about available platforms and try one or more before making a final choice.

EndNote and Mendeley are similar programs for managing your citations. EndNote is available for macOS and Windows, while Mendeley is available for macOS, Windows, and Linux. EndNote offers a basic web-based version that is free, although many universities offer access to the full version for their students. Mendeley offers free access to their program but requires registration. Both EndNote and Mendeley offer limited online storage of references for free, and their premium/paid versions offer greatly increased storage. Both EndNote and Mendeley (free and paid) offer plugins to allow you to "cite while you write" in Microsoft Word for both macOS and Windows. You can find out more about EndNote and Mendeley by visiting their respective websites.

PaperPile is a browser-based citation-management system that is integrated fully with Google Drive and Google Docs. It offers a free 30-day trial and an academic discount to students. PaperPile is the only available citation manager for users who want to "cite while they write" in Google Docs. It requires the use of Google's Chrome browser.

Papers is a reference-management software that is available only on macOS. It has a plugin to allow "cite while you write" within Word for macOS. Find out more about PaperPile and Papers online.

ORAL DEFENSE

When the PhD thesis is submitted to the university, the next phase is the oral defense. The purpose of the oral defense is to ensure that the PhD candidate can present and defend their thesis and effectively communicate their important work to the community. Two important tasks to complete before the defense can take place are to form an oral defense committee and to schedule the oral defense. The defense committee requirements vary by school. For example, Johns Hopkins University requires five committee members. Harvard University requires that three or four Harvard faculty members serve on the committee. McGill University requires a five-member committee, unless three of these members have been closely involved with the thesis, in which case a seven-member committee is required. For the University of Toronto, the thesis examination committee requires a quorum of at least four members. For most schools, each committee member other than an external member must hold a faculty position at the university.

The committee members include a non-voting chairperson appointed by the school or department, the thesis supervisor(s), an internal examiner, and at least one external committee member. The internal examiner is a faculty member of the university who has not been affiliated with the research project, while the external committee member cannot be a faculty member of the department/faculty of the student.

The exact format of the oral defense presentation is different at each university. For example, Johns Hopkins University does not have a time requirement, while Harvard University recommends an hour for the presentation. McGill University requires that the student present for 20 minutes, while the University of British Columbia allots a maximum of 30 minutes. However, the presentation has common requirements across universities: it should focus on the original contributions that the PhD thesis makes to the field.

Following the presentation, a question-and-answer session will take place that may last an hour and a half or longer. A PhD oral defense usually lasts at least two hours, including the presentation and questions. The questions are asked by the oral defense committee and will usually be asked in rounds. The response to individual questions should be brief and to the point. The questions should mainly focus on the thesis but may also test the candidate's background knowledge. Following one or more rounds of questions from the oral defense committee members, the thesis chairperson may open the floor to questions from the audience.

After the question-and-answer period is concluded, the audience and candidate must leave the room for a private evaluation session that may last up to 50 minutes. During this evaluation session, the oral defense committee will determine whether the thesis meets the academic standards for a PhD dissertation, the candidate demonstrated the ability to effectively communicate and defend their work, and the candidate possesses sufficient knowledge and understanding of the field.

The outcome of the oral defense will be communicated to the candidate after the evaluation period. The evaluation will usually be in the form of a pass or a fail. In case of a failure, the evaluation may offer to allow the candidate to conduct another oral defense within a set time frame (e.g., six months) or to submit a revised thesis within a similar time frame.

TIPS FOR A SUCCESSFUL PRESENTATION AND QUESTION-AND-ANSWER SESSION

Putting together a brief, coherent scientific presentation is an art form. I've been told by seasoned academics that they are still working on improving their presentation skills. Students should expect and actively seek out constructive criticism from their supervisor(s), other students, and thesis committee members. As practice makes perfect, students should also practice their presentation multiple times and in front of different people. For additional presentation strategies and advice, students should carefully read Chapter 17 on networking and presentations as an MD-PhD student.

For the question-and-answer session, preparation is key. Students should remember that when they are at this stage in their program, they are the expert on the topic and project. Careful anticipation of potential questions can allow the student to prepare slides on anticipated topics beforehand. I often adopt this strategy and have slides at the end of my presentation available to address difficult concepts or questions. Often, just going through the process of preparing an introductory slide helps me to review and solidify these topics in my mind and negates their need; however, having a visual on the topics can demonstrate careful planning to the committee.

During the session, make sure to always smile and be polite. When a question is asked, it can be useful to clarify the question by repeating it back to the questioner in your own words. Only once you completely understand the question should a response to the question be made. Before answering the question, a polite comment should be made to the questioner, such as, "That is an excellent question, thank you for asking." Remember that you are not expected to know everything; it is perfectly acceptable to admit this and to acknowledge that you will have to read more about the topic. Also remember to think carefully before responding. It is acceptable to make a statement such as, "Please give me a moment to think about this question."

Posture and body language are also important. Make sure to stand up straight and maintain eye contact with your audience and questioners. Even if heated questions are asked, make sure to be friendly and warm, as smiling and polite responses will keep your question-and-answer session as relaxed as possible. Lastly, remember to breathe and to take your time. Speak slowly and think carefully before responding.

CONCLUSION

Writing a doctoral thesis is a stressful and time-consuming process. To facilitate this process, remember to follow your school's specific guidelines for the structure of your thesis, write early and often, choose (and learn to use) a citation-management software, and keep your reference list up-to-date (starting from your initial literature review). Finally, don't neglect yourself. Make time for friends, family, and fun and stay active.

17

Networking as MD-PhD Students

Tianwei Ellen Zhou

Tianwei Ellen Zhou *obtained her BSc, MD, and PhD degrees from McGill University. She is pursuing her ophthalmology residency at Université de Montréal. Her research focuses on retinopathy of prematurity (ROP), a blinding eye disease that affects many premature infants.*

INTRODUCTION

"The future is today," Sir William Osler once said. In medicine as in networking. Our connections today came from the like-minded people we met in the past. And new friendships stem from people we meet today and in the future. If your goal is to excel in your MD-PhD studies, having a health network is the icing on the cake.

WE ARE ALL INTERDEPENDENT

Everyone plays a role in your career. When I was a new graduate student in the laboratory, I asked questions frequently, from troubleshooting western blots to navigating the convoluted ethics' board approval. I learned tremendously from laboratory technicians who had 20 years of experience in molecular biology. To ask relevant questions rather than trivial ones, it is important to do some independent research beforehand.

As I became a more senior member in the lab, I was able to pay back and pass down experiences to my junior colleagues—teaching culturing techniques for a difficult cell line, training new members on subretinal injections for small rodents, and sharing my thoughts on preparing a successful committee meeting. We also helped each other when some members were absent from the lab. I tended cells (and pet plants) and inspected equipment during Christmas and New Year. Similarly, my colleagues fed my mice when I was away. To this date, even after I graduated from my doctoral training, my colleagues

WHAT YOU NEED TO KNOW

- Be friendly—everyone can teach you something.
- Pay it forward and help others.
- Find your support groups.
- Go to conferences and talk to people.
- Spend some time managing your LinkedIn profile.

and I still meet from time to time, updating each other on our lives. My lab mates were an important part in my graduate study. Now, my present and future colleagues are just as indispensable.

A SUPPORT GROUP AND AN ADVISORY BOARD

There is no doubt that your 7–8 years of MD-PhD training are filled with challenges. There will be times that you are juggling experiments, manuscript writing, and preparation for your final exams. Networking and forming a support group with your fellow MD-PhD classmates are helpful. That is because you all are going through the same process, understanding each other. Go grab a dinner with them, and talk about the challenges you are facing.

Sharing your experiences does not only ease the anxiety, but also allows you to come up with a solution as a group. For example, when you are struggling to write a competitive scholarship application, feel free to reach out to a senior member in your program and ask for advice. Your supervisor may have assigned you a cool research project, but a successful scholarship application takes more than something cool. Your classmates can emphasize to the importance of extracurricular activities, leadership engagement, and volunteer experiences. In McGill's MD-PhD program, we invited our senior students and graduates who had recently gone through clerkship, electives, and the Canadian Resident Matching Service (CaRMS) to pass their experiences to the juniors.

EXPLORING FUTURE OPPORTUNITIES AND FORMING FUTURE ALLIANCES

Have you considered that the graduate students and MD-PhD classmates you are working with now can be your future collaborators? There is an increasing trend in North America that a grant application requires a team of investigators. Such team is often multidisciplinary, including basic scientists, clinician-investigators, engineers, and more.

The PhD/MSc students you meet during your graduate study may well turn into your long-term collaborators in the future. Take Simon for example. I met him during my PhD. He was the new graduate student in the neighboring lab, which was also relatively new. Simon wore thick glasses and always told me, with a genuine excitement, about his work on optical coherence tomography (OCT). Being in the field of vision science, I had used OCT before; it is a noninvasive machine that gives a quick scan of the retina. OCT works like an ultrasound (no radiation), except that it offers a much higher resolution. In the past decade, it has quickly become a powerful research and diagnostic tool in ophthalmology.

During lunch time, we chatted about our research projects. He told me about the engineering aspect of an OCT machine, which involved PhD-level math and engineering—knowledge that is outside my scope of training. Nonetheless, I was impressed by his knowledge and the plan to improve this technology. Fast-forwarding to my residency, my research project needed a special kind of OCT with a tailored lens. I immediately thought of Simon and proposed to my research mentor a collaboration with him and his supervisor. We soon met with both teams and had an insightful conversation. Eventually, a new project unfolded. That collaboration was first forged during those nonchalant lunch conversations.

JUST HAVE A CONVERSATION

Just like the many lunch conversations with Simon, networking comes naturally: Simply talk to people and get to know them (not at the expense of your productivity, of course). Post-docs, summer interns, electricians, unit coordinators, head nurses, and cleaning staff—all make a contribution to the daily running of a laboratory or a hospital unit. They can teach us something valuable. When I was working in an old research building, an electrician once told me that there were occasional power outages at night. These power outages briefly shut off cell incubators and reset the temperature sensor. Thinking that could be the reason for the loss of our precious cell lines, we moved all incubators to an adjacent building with a stable power supply. No cells were ever again lost due to fluctuating temperatures.

JOIN STUDENT GROUPS

Student groups are fun and are good support systems. I have met many inspiring people by participating in them. They have shown me different ways and directions to develop my career. They are also an opportunity to keep in touch with both aspects of your future as a physician-scientist, and are one possible avenue through which to maintain clinical skills during PhD training (Chapter 14).

I had been a long-term executive member of the Clinician-Investigator Trainee Association of Canada (CITAC), the national student body for Canadian MD-PhD trainees. Each year, CITAC organizes annual meetings (often in Toronto), when most of the MD-PhD trainees from coast to coast meet. We compared our curricula, funding sources, mentorship opportunities, and administrative support. We realized that though our curricula were similar, Canadian MD-PhD programs differed in many important aspects. One may think administrative support is a trivial matter (or simply peripherally related to the scientific endeavor). I soon learned that at one school, medical students were reluctant to pursue the MD-PhD path because they had to jump through administrative hoops without support. They mentioned the lack of a centralized office that helped them transition between graduate study and medical school, and the absence of a medical curriculum which accommodates independent research time.

Later on, I shared this observation with our program director, Dr. Mark Eisenberg. I expressed my surprise at learning students would forgo a career path because no one was helping with the paperwork. Intrigued by what makes a conducive and productive MD-PhD program, we embarked on a project that examined the strengths and weakness of McGill's own program. With Paul Savage, a fellow MD-PhD student (and now a general surgery resident at University of Toronto), we carried out an alumni survey for all McGill graduates in the past 30 years. We eventually published our findings in a peer-reviewed paper, reaching out to a wide readership. Based on suggestions from our alumni, Dr. Eisenberg implemented several new changes, including streamlining the administrative process to facilitate graduate school-medical school transition. The idea of conducting this survey could be traced to a conference conversation. But it was the collaborative teamwork that resulted in tangible improvements. During this process, I had the opportunity to work closely with MD-PhD program directors, classmates, alumni, and staff from the faculty of medicine. We formed strong bonds as colleagues and friends over meetings, discussion, and sometimes over dinners. Now that I have started my residency, I still keep in touch with many of them.

GO TO CONFERENCES AND PRESENT YOUR WORK

Conferences, especially international ones, are wonderful opportunities to showcase your work and to network broadly. Take the CITAC annual meeting for example. Trainees from different backgrounds—MD-PhD students, clinical investigator program (CIP) trainees, research fellows, and MD-PhD representatives from the United States—get together and chat about basically anything. It is a meeting where you can learn about how different MD-PhD programs work in Canada and the United States.

In addition, CITAC meetings also offer professional development workshops. Take the 2016 conference for example. At lunchtime, they invited physician-scientists from different subspecialties (psychiatry, general surgery, and internal medicine, for instance) to chat about how to coordinate clinical duty and research. Trainees were welcome to rotate between tables so that they could have diverse perspectives. There were also multiple afternoon boot camps on grant writing, manuscript preparation, salary negotiation, equity and diversity, and applying for academic jobs. Trainees chose the ones appropriate to their level of training and personal interests. We often saw premed students, pondering if an MD-PhD was right for them, attending CITAC meetings and asking questions.

Besides national and regional events, international conferences are important as they foster broad collaboration and facilitate your career transition. Posters and oral presentations are great ways to be known by others, and going to other people's posters and oral presentations and asking questions helps you get to know people, too. This is particularly relevant when you are applying to your residency or fellowship positions. Bigger meetings also create the opportunity for social events; they are lighthearted occasions to see old friends and make new ones.

THE POWER OF SOCIAL MEDIA

In the past 10 years, social media has become an indispensable means for networking. It can diversify and expand one's network, strength weak ties, and nurture longtime relationships. In this chapter, I focus the discussion on four common social media outlets—Twitter, Facebook, LinkedIn, and Instagram—for networking purpose (rather than personal use).

Twitter

I endorse Twitter because it is succinct. With a few words, you can deliver a great deal of information, all thanks to hashtags. For example, when I share an article, I describe the research in a few words and provide a link to the original website plus #science (or #ophthalmology if applicable). Because #science is quite a popular topic at the time of the tweet, it has a substantially broader reach to other people, even those who aren't your followers. Thousands of people who click on that hashtag every hour around the world might see it, providing extra exposure to your post. Similar, during our annual general meetings at CITAC, we encouraged attendees to use #citacagm to advertise the event and reach out to those who could not attend in person.

LinkedIn

LinkedIn is my social media of preference when it comes to networking. I like it for its professionalism, with a focus on work rather than personal life. I use LinkedIn to connect with colleagues whom I meet in conferences or from work. (Facebook and Instagram are for my personal life. But you can nonetheless create accounts on behalf of your group or organization.) Many websites provide sound recommendations on how to use LinkedIn, and a quick online search can offer plenty of advice for you to consider when creating your profile.

Besides creating a solid profile, there are plenty of practices that can make your networking experience on LinkedIn more effective and rewarding. Many of my LinkedIn contacts have asked for recommendations (likely during their career transitions), to testify to their professionalism or to endorse their technical expertise. Most of the time I agreed to do so as long as I had worked with them and what they asked was founded. Everyone needs a bit of help in their careers; paying it forward always paves the way for your future self when help is needed.

Most importantly, be present. Many people create an account and leave it dormant. I suggest logging in at least once a week to see if someone has sent you a friend request or contacted you via the built-in mailing system. When your contacts have a work anniversary or publish an interesting article, pressing a little like button or saying congratulations is quite heartwarming. For people whom you know well or for a long time, dropping a short message goes a long way.

CONCLUSION

A broad network does not come overnight. It takes effort to foster new connections and maintain existing ones. Thanks to new technologies and social media, we have more networking tools at our disposal than before. They have helped us to keep track of friends' life events: birthdays, status updates, and developments. Don't be shy to write them a little message on their special days; kind gestures like this go a long way.

At the same time, traditional means of networking, such as conferences and interest groups, still play a critical role. In fact, I found that face-to-face conversation is the most powerful and effective way to get to know a person. Grabbing a coffee with someone you knew from online networking is extremely helpful to create a stronger professional relationship.

Ultimately, as you put yourself into other people's shoes, you would want to meet someone who is positive, passionate, polite, and honest. So be that likable person. Lastly, it is never too late to create your network. "The future is today". Your network in two months depends on what you are doing today.

Part IV

Transitioning Back to Medical School

18

Preparing for Your Return to the Wards

Shira G. Ziegler

Shira G, Ziegler *graduated from The Johns Hopkins University School of Medicine MD-PhD program in 2018. Her graduate research elucidated the mechanisms underlying rare disorders of ectopic calcification and identified potential treatment strategies. She is currently pursuing dual residency training in pediatrics and medical genetics at The Johns Hopkins Hospital and plans to combine her bench-to-bedside research on rare genetic conditions with clinical care. Prior to medical school, Shira graduated from Oberlin College with highest honors in neuroscience and worked in the National Institutes of Health's Undiagnosed Diseases Program and Human Genome Research Institute.*

INTRODUCTION

Many MD-PhD students are concerned about the transition back to medical school after their graduate studies. It is a justifiable concern. You have just spent the last 3–6 years becoming an expert in your field of research, and now you have to return to medical school, with medical students who were likely in high school when you started your medical training and, residents and fellows who were previously your peers. In addition, while you have spent the past number of years honing your technical and analytical skills, you have understandably forgotten some of the underlying pathology and pathophysiology, in addition to clinical skills, learned during the first 2 years of medical school. Chapter 14 of this book presented tips on maintaining your clinical skills and knowledge in graduate school. However, most MD-PhD students take Step 1 of the United States Medical Licensing Exam (Chapter 21, USMLE) before pursuing graduate training and do not have another opportunity for a systematic review of the preclinical material before embarking on their clinical clerkships.

WHAT YOU NEED TO KNOW

- Register for re-matriculation early.
- Aim to reenter the medical school curriculum in the summer or early fall of the equivalent to the third year of medical studies.
- If time permits, participate in a clerkship or shadowing in the year prior to re-matriculation.
- Get recertified/re-credentialed where it is required several months before your return.
- Rediscover old skills, resources, and equipment, and discover new ones in the month before your return to medical school.

While this transition is challenging, planning and organization can help ease reintegration into the medical school curriculum.

CHOOSING YOUR RE-MATRICULATION DATE

At least 1 year before you anticipate going back to the wards, it is crucial that you talk to your institution's registrar. For most institutions, there are only certain times when MD-PhD students can reenter the curriculum. The institution's annual master academic schedule is usually determined 1–2 years in advance, so the potential reentry points should be clear. For maximum efficiency, MD-PhDs should try to reenter the medical school curriculum in the summer or early fall of the equivalent to their third year of medical studies. The earlier you register, the more likely you will get your preferred core clerkship and elective schedule (refer to chapter 19 for more details). If your plans change, with the most likely scenario that your PhD research and manuscript are taking longer than anticipated, you can usually defer reentry for another year, though make sure to let your registrar know with adequate warning. If you are uncertain of your exact timeline, it is much easier to plan for re-matriculation and potentially defer instead of scrambling at the last minute to find open clerkship slots.

Students can strategically enter the clinical curriculum earlier or later depending on their timeline and objectives. If a student enters earlier, there is typically more free time for clinical exploration in the form of electives. This is helpful if a student is uncertain about their clinical interests. With additional time, there is also the possibility of interspersing your third and fourth years of medical school with research electives to complete lingering experiments or reviews on a manuscript. While it is highly suggested, and likely required, that you finish all PhD requirements before re-matriculating in medical school, sometimes the timing is simply inopportune. For example, there are situations in which it makes more sense to go back to medical school for two to four months of clinical clerkships while a manuscript is out for review and then return for a one-month research elective to finish the manuscript. You should discuss this in detail with your MD-PhD program director and principal investigator (PI) before pursuing this path. Re-matriculation can also occur later in the academic year if a student is confident in their clinical interests or a decision not to pursue a clinical residency after graduation.

It is essential that you understand the clinical and elective requirements at your institution. For most MD-PhD programs, the PhD years count toward some but usually not all of the elective requirements. Some curriculums are more lenient with elective requirements than others. Choose a re-matriculation date that allows you to schedule all the necessary clinical and elective requirements. Also, plan your schedule strategically; remember that clinical grades after September of your fourth year of medical school will not display on your transcript to residency programs. Ensure that there is enough time to do one or two sub-internships and electives—either at your institution or as an away elective—to help narrow your clinical interests and strengthen your residency application.

PRE-RETURN COMMITMENTS: TIMELINE

In the year before you return to the wards, your focus should be on completing your PhD thesis and manuscripts, as addressed in Chapter 15 ("Completing Your Project") and Chapter 16 ("Thesis Writing"). If time permits, there are usually opportunities for MD-PhD students to participate in a year-long longitudinal clerkship in preparation for the transition back to the wards. Most of these opportunities occur weekly in the primary care setting to help re-familiarize students with the physical exam and common disease pathologies. For a less formal long-term commitment, you can consider shadowing opportunities in clinics of interest. You can also attend department-specific grand rounds. Reread Chapter 14 to explore ways to stay connected to clinical medicine throughout your graduate school training.

Three months before you go back to medical school, it is a good idea to start your re-certification process. Contact your MD-PhD program administrators and registrar's office to determine the requirements. Most MD-PhD students' Basic Life Safety (BLS) certification will have lapsed during their graduate studies. Most institutions require that you recertify before starting on the clinical wards. In addition, you will likely need to be re-credentialed into your instituition's electronic medical record (EMR) system. This will likely require online training or learning modules focused on patient privacy and confidentiality. Once re-credentialed in the EMR, take time to familiarize yourself with the software. Specifically, determine where to find vitals, orders, laboratory values, and how to read and write notes. Talk to more senior MD-PhD colleagues about the standard note templates used on different clerkships. Since most of your time as a medical student is spent pre-charting, seeing patients, and writing notes, strong familiarity with the EMR will make this process much easier.

Within one month of returning to the wards, see if you can take advantage of an opportunity to work with a standardized patient to review a full head-to-toe physical exam. Not only is this important to refresh your physical exam skills, but it is also necessary to know the precise exam maneuvers that will be expected during future clinical skills training exams that are common during third and fourth year of medical school.

The month before returning to the wards is also an opportunity to determine the clinical resources you plan on using during your clerkships. Many medical students rely on question banks and review books to study for shelf exams. Consider purchasing a 1- or 2-year question bank subscription to use throughout the rest of your clinical years and to study for Step 2 of the United States Medical Licensing Exam (USMLE). Many senior MD-PhD students have books, either hard copy or electronic, that they are happy to share. This is also a good time to reconnect with the clinical advisor assigned to you during your pre-clinical years. There is a chance that your clinical advisor might have left the position. If so, ask your dean's office for a new assignment. Your clinical advisor will be an invaluable resource as you navigate through your clerkships and prepare to apply for residency.

Evaluate your financial situation and consider taking out loans. There are numerous expenses generated during your last year of medical school, such as those for residency interviews (Chapter 22). Depending on your MD-PhD program's structure, you might be eligible for different loans during graduate school compared to medical school. Sometimes it is advantageous to take out loans during your graduate training. If so, make sure the appropriate paperwork is complete before transitioning back to medical school. Talk to your financial aid office for more information and advice.

Finally, find your white coat and stethoscope! If you cannot find your white coat, or if it is not so white anymore after hiding in the back of your closet, consider purchasing a new one or getting it professionally cleaned.

CONCLUSION

Overall, even though the transition back to the wards is daunting, MD-PhD students usually excel. With years of additional experience, training, and maturity, MD-PhD students tend to relate more easily not only to their patients but also to the provider teams. MD-PhD trainees should be confident in their transition back to medical school and excited about entering the final 2 years of training. The marathon's end is in sight.

19

Strategic Selection of Rotations and Electives

Paul Savage

Paul Savage *graduated from the MD-PhD program at McGill University in 2019. His research focused on mechanisms of drug sensitivity in breast cancer, using patient-derived tumor models. He then pursued residency training in general surgery at the University of Toronto.*

INTRODUCTION

Core rotations and electives are designed not only to broaden and enhance your knowledge base across the various disciplines of medicine, but also to give you opportunities to explore specialties you might pursue as a career. Generally speaking, the choices discussed in this chapter are made around the same time as you are returning to the wards (Chapter 18, Preparing for Your Return to the Wards) and will impact your future choice of residency (Chapter 22, Choosing the Right Residency, Applying, and Interviewing). Strategies for selecting rotations and electives have long been passed down by word-of-mouth from more senior medical trainees. These are naturally largely anecdotal, with no single approach being foolproof. Here, we discuss some of these strategies in general, as well as some special considerations for MD-PhD students.

FINDING YOUR FUTURE SPECIALTY

While many MD-PhD trainees develop areas of clinical interest related to the topic of their doctoral studies, this is not always the case. The reality is that most research subjects are approached clinically through multidisciplinary teams and can therefore be addressed through

WHAT YOU NEED TO KNOW

- Exposure to the field in question is key when picking a medical specialty.
- Elective strategies are highly personalized. Spend time reflecting on your own values.
- Start the process early and respect deadlines.
- Don't stress; nobody has the perfect rotation stream or elective schedule.
- Take all advice (including this) with a grain of salt.

careers across a multitude of specialties. For example, if you are interested in mechanisms of chronic pain, you may develop clinical interests in anesthesia, neurology, psychiatry, or family medicine. If your PhD was focused on pediatric brain tumors, you may consider pursuing neurosurgery, pediatric hematology-oncology, or radiation oncology. While the theory of a given topic may pique your curiosity, you need to be passionate about the day-to-day medical practice to develop a sustainable career as a physician-scientist. A large proportion of MD-PhD students end up finding clinical interests outside of their PhD research field, which they decide to further pursue in residency. Your doctoral training provides you with a transferable skill set that can be adapted to many fields and should not limit you to specific specialties.

The factors that influence your decision in specialization are highly individualized and covered in Chapter 22. Some of the reasons to consider a given specialty include the types of patient encounters, the patient population, the acuity of illness, whether there is a surgical/procedural component, the feasibility of developing a parallel research program, lifestyle, competitiveness of matching to residency positions, and future employment opportunities and earning potential. Classically, one of the first branch points many trainees decide on is medical versus surgical specialties.

Exposure is essential when choosing a clinical career. While pre-clerkship shadowing, special interest groups, and mentors may provide early direction, it is mostly through your core rotations and electives where you will identify and further solidify your clinical interests. It is important to remain objective during this process and continuously reflect on your values. Find a field that makes you excited to go in each morning. Do not fall for the prestige of the surgeon if you cannot stand being in the operating room as your case extends into the middle of the night. Ask yourself whether you could work with these colleagues, but remember that you can easily be swayed toward or away from a specialty by a single experience with a good or bad team. This is why developing a personalized strategy to rotations and electives is an important step in your development as a physician-scientist.

The more immediate implications of strategizing electives involve your residency application. With increasing competitiveness of most residency programs, many applicants will decide whether they are more willing to compromise on geographic location of program or on their residency specialty. Weighing these factors should help guide your overall elective strategy.

CORE ROTATIONS

It is during your core rotations when you really start refining the list of specialties you are considering applying to for residency. As opposed to electives, third-year core rotations are for the most part standardized, and there is little room for strategy. Having said that, there are a few considerations when organizing your core rotations.

How should I pick my core rotation stream?

At some medical schools, you may be able to rank the order of your core rotation stream. If you are unsure of what you want to do exactly but have one or two specialties in mind, it is ideal to have these core blocks between October and January of your third year. This will give you the time to adapt to the clinical setting during your first couple of rotations, so by this point you will be well-adjusted and able to make a positive impression. Additionally, if you find that the rotation confirmed your interest in the field, you will have ample time to begin setting up fourth-year electives. On the other hand, if you realize you are no longer interested in that field, you have ample time to begin planning alternative strategies for your electives.

Another important point about ranking your stream is that some schools have mandatory core rotations or electives in the fourth year. While you'll be focusing much of your energy on excelling during your electives, putting time into your residency application is equally important. It can be challenging to do both exceptionally well, which is why scheduling a light block in the month or two preceding these application deadlines can be a good idea. The alternative is using a vacation block.

What should I do my selectives/subspecialty rotations in?

Many schools require subspecialty selectives (e.g., internal medicine, pediatrics, or surgery) as part of the core curriculum, which can be in either third or fourth year. If one of these happens to be your first-choice discipline, you should treat it like an elective at your home school. For example, if you are aiming for general surgery, a selective in a general surgery subspecialty (e.g., trauma surgery or thoracic surgery) is more useful for your application than orthopedics or plastic surgery.

How should I approach my core rotations?

When it comes to performance during core rotations, it is best to approach each core rotation as if this is what you are applying to. Not only will this make you a more balanced physician, it will result in better evaluations on your record, which provide a strong safety net should you end up deciding to pursue a different field than you anticipated. It is also important to develop good habits during your core rotations. Showing up every day with a positive attitude, being a team player (with interdisciplinary professionals, residents, and other medical students), taking initiative and ownership in your daily work, knowing your limitations, asking thoughtful questions, and developing a study plan will carry you a long way. Constantly put yourself in the shoes of the junior resident and try to anticipate the decisions they face every day. Showing off these features will demonstrate that you are trustworthy, safe, and teachable, features that make excellent residents.

ELECTIVES

The increasingly competitive nature of residency matching has led to a culture where many medical students stack all of their electives in a single discipline. While trainees see this as a way to demonstrate their commitment to a given specialty and network with potential residency programs, it goes against the primary objective of electives, which is to develop well-rounded medical graduates who have informed their career trajectories through diverse exposure to medical specialties. While Americans can still choose to do the majority of their electives within a single discipline, the Association of Faculties of Medicine of Canada (AFMC) has developed an elective diversification policy, which states that "student elective opportunities cannot exceed a maximum of eight weeks in any single entry-level discipline."* This has been unanimously adopted by all Canadian medical schools beginning for the class of 2021. Considering this, here are several questions MD-PhD trainees may ask as they approach clerkship.

---

*An entry-level discipline is an Entry Route in the PGY-1 (R1) Match. Each of these entry-level disciplines leads to specialty certification with either the Royal College of Physicians and Surgeons of Canada (RCPSC) or the Certification in the College of Family Physicians (CCFP). Electives in subspecialties that are part of a PGY-3 (R3) match (such as the subspecialties in Internal Medicine and Pediatrics) are counted as separate disciplines. As such, electives in these subspecialties do not count toward the eight-week maximum in the general specialty.

When should I start planning my electives?

Organizing visiting electives requires meticulous planning and a firm understanding of the application process. Some schools accept elective applications through a centralized portal, such as the Association of American Medical Colleges (AAMC) or the AFMC, while others require direct institutional applications. This leads to variability in terms of timing of elective planning, yet there are some general recommendations that can be made. Begin arranging documents, including your resume, immunization record, mask-fitting documentation, a headshot, and a police check seven to eight months prior to your first elective. Other documentations that you may require, particularly if applying in the United States, include a dean's letter, Test of English as a Foreign Language (TOEFL) and United States Medical Licensing Examination (USMLE) Step 1 exam results, Health Insurance Portability and Accountability (HIPAA) certification, cardiopulmonary resuscitation/basic life support (CPR/BLS) certification, and professional liability/malpractice and health insurance. Most schools start accepting applications 26 weeks (six and a half months) prior to the start date. If you are applying to highly sought-after electives, your application will need to be submitted on the earliest day possible. You may be able to apply to electives at your home school with a little more flexibility. Some students who are undecided on a given specialty or location decide to double-book electives (two or more separate electives confirmed during a single time period) so that they can defer their elective choice when they are more certain of what they want. While it is technically allowed if all but one elective are cancelled on time (usually six to eight weeks prior to the start date), this approach is costly to students, unprofessional, and a burden to administrators, and therefore should be discouraged.

What should I do for my third-year elective?

If you are fairly certain of what specialty you want to apply for by the beginning of clerkship, use your third year elective to confirm your interest in that field. Because you have likely had very limited if any clinical experience in this field, you do not want to do it at your first-choice school. One strategy would be to do your third-year elective at your home school, where you may be comfortable with the clinical setting (e.g., hospital, electronic medical record) and can focus on gaining a better understanding of the routine pathologies you will be coming across during the rest of your visiting electives in this field. If you are still undecided on what specialty you would like to pursue, the third-year elective is the key time to get exposure to these fields.

How long should I schedule each elective?

Electives are offered in two-, three-, or four-week blocks, each of which has its own advantages and disadvantages. Shorter (two-week) electives allow you to visit multiple places. However, it can be a challenge to adapt to the new environment and make a lasting impression within the short time frame. Longer electives (four weeks) allow you to become quite comfortable within a given field at a specific location. However, it can be a bit of a risk in case you don't click with the team. While three-week electives are a nice balance, they pose a logistical challenge in terms of scheduling, because of the way periods are organized into four-week time frames. For this reason, you might consider doing longer electives at one or two schools you think you will rank highly and shorter electives at a few schools that you think will fall lower on your list. You will also likely want to do two-week electives for those specialties that are not your first choice.

Where should I do my electives?

Few if any programs explicitly require you to do an elective at their site to get an interview, though you should review this in the program descriptions at the school-specific Electronic Residency Application Service (ERAS) and/or Canadian Resident Matching Service (CaRMS) websites. You may hear of certain programs in which there is an unwritten requirement to do an elective at their school, but these are highly unpredictable and should not necessarily sway your elective strategy. If you are aiming for a specific specialty and willing to compromise on location, a reasonable approach is to do one elective at your home school, and others scattered across the country. Not only will this demonstrate your willingness to move, but a reference letter from a familiar colleague may have more of an impact. You may also have the opportunity to do rural or urban electives within your specialty of interest at a given school. While rural electives may offer more hands-on experience and a great learning experience, the program committees are generally located at the main sites of the medical school. Therefore, doing all your electives at remote sites would not be advisable. Similarly, if you are interested in doing your residency in another country, then you should plan on doing several electives in that country. However, if you are planning on applying through ERAS or CaRMS, you should do the overwhelming majority of your electives within the United States or Canada.

How should I order my electives?

One of the main factors to consider when selecting the order of your electives is the deadlines for residency applications and providing sufficient time for your referees to write your letters of reference. Because it will strengthen your application, you should do your electives and get letters from your top-choice schools prior to these deadlines. Again, doing an elective at your home institution may ease the challenges with adapting to a new environment, which is why doing this elective first may be helpful. If your home institution is your top choice, then you might consider doing this elective a little later. You will want to have completed a few weeks in your specialty before doing an elective at your top-choice program so that you are very comfortable with the routine cases and perform as best as you can. Many choose to leave their electives in other disciplines until after the application deadline. Do not worry if this is not possible and you are only able to get an elective at a specific program in your top-choice specialty after application deadline, as your presence on the service during the application review process may play out in your favor, because evaluators will not have a chance to forget who you are.

Apart from my first-choice discipline, what other fields should I do electives in?

Most medical schools require students to do at least two weeks of electives across at least three parental disciplines (e.g., internal medicine, pediatrics, general surgery, etc). It's important to know your own medical school's policy to properly plan these electives, which you can find online or through the career counselor. This means you need to think about electives in other disciplines that will strengthen your application to your first-choice specialty. There are many elective combinations that naturally complement each other. For example, if you are interested in emergency medicine, you might consider doing electives in anesthesiology to work on your airway management and line access, trauma surgery to familiarize yourself with your trauma survey, or diagnostic radiology to improve your X-ray interpretation. If you find yourself interested in dermatology, you can work on your procedural skills during a plastic surgery elective, refine your pathology, and/or refresh yourself on classic exanthems by spending time with infectious disease. If you enjoy working with children and are considering a subspecialty of pediatrics, it's important to know the entry-level program (e.g., pediatric rheumatology via pediatrics versus pediatric neurosurgery via neurosurgery), as you will want to plan your electives accordingly. There are certain fields, often those which we may have little exposure to in medical school, which can complement essentially any application, including radiology and critical care. Remember that nontraditional electives can also be used to diversify your application, and include fields like medical education, global health, or research.

Can I select a specific supervisor for my elective?

With the centralization of elective applications through AAMC/AFMC, many schools no longer allow you to select a specific supervisor you would like to work with. At the remaining schools that do allow you to directly contact potential supervisors, find someone whose letter will carry weight. These people are not necessarily program directors but may be closely involved in residency education, whether it be a program committee member, a prominent member of the department, or a division chief. Even if you cannot spend your full elective with one of these individuals, seek out any opportunity to interact with them, whether by doing a day in clinic with them or spending an afternoon in their operating room. If your senior resident sees you working hard on your elective and is aware of your interest in their program, they will often try to maximize your exposure with these important staff members.

Should I do a research elective?

Since you are an MD-PhD student, research electives are certainly not a requirement to match to a competitive specialty. By the time you reach clerkship, you likely have done far more research than the majority of your peers. While doing a formal research elective may not be necessary, pursuing research projects in your spare time allows you to explore your clinical interest in more depth and develop working relationships with individuals involved in residency programs you are interested in. If you plan on doing visiting electives, consider doing portable research, such as a systematic review or clinical studies where a database already exists. A publication or conference presentation within your clinical domain will undoubtedly enhance your residency application.

Should I parallel plan with another specialty?

After you pick your first-choice specialty, decide whether you will parallel plan or back up is one of the most difficult decisions you will make during clerkship. Some people who are torn between two competitive specialties decide to go for both, which should theoretically be facilitated by the AFMC elective diversification policy. If this is what you decide to do, you must have some well-constructed answers for why you are fully committed to two different specialties by the time residency interviews arrive (Chapter 22). Others decide to go all in on a single specialty without any alternatives. Some back up with less competitive specialties (e.g., family medicine). There is no universal answer to this challenging problem. At the very least, if you are not willing to back up, you should be prepared to go to a geographic area that is not your first choice. Conversely, if you are set on a specific city, you have to accept that you may not get into your top specialty. You ultimately need to feel comfortable with your final rank list, including the possibility of going unmatched should you decide not to back up. Finally, do not feel locked into a given specialty. If you realize that you are not built to be an orthopedic surgeon after a couple electives, it's never too late to change your mind. Once you identify this might be the case, however, gather support from your career counseling office as early as possible so that you can begin re-strategizing.

How should I budget for electives?

Electives add to the cost of your final year of medical school and should be factored into your budget. This includes registration with AAMC and/or AFMC and application fees as well as cost of travel and accommodations during your visiting electives. Some of these can be reduced by medical association travel/accommodation deals, staying with friends/family, or at university residences. Additional costs will be incurred later in your fourth year, such as ERAS/CaRMS application fees, travel and accommodations expenses during interviews, licensing exam registration fees, and costs of moving to your new residency program. While these amounts seem significant as a trainee, you should not base your residency application decisions on them, and financial planners will be easily accessible to help you set up a responsible budget for your final year.

What should I be doing while on elective?

In addition to the work ethic you have developed during your core rotations, there are a few extra things that you'll want to do while on elective in your first-choice specialty. Spend the weekend before your rotation reviewing the common topics you'll be encountering during your elective. Stay later the first few evenings of your rotation, reviewing the charts of your inpatients so you know their history and disease course, and read up on patients you will be seeing in the following day's clinic or operating room. Take as much call as you can, particularly if it is with your senior resident. Not only will you get better exposure during the night when fewer residents are around, but your senior resident may advocate for you when admission decisions are being made. Be flexible and proactive. If another service is short a resident, offer to help out so long as it does not hurt your own team. Try to present at departmental rounds. Ask for constructive midway and end-of-rotation feedback, specifying concrete steps that you can take to become a better trainee. On the last day of your rotation, find the staff whom you have worked closest with and ask for a letter of reference in person, while providing them with an updated resume and draft of your personal letter. Some people also decide to meet individually with program directors during their visiting electives, but only do this if you genuinely have questions, as you will likely be the person guiding the conversation. Lastly, it can be difficult to keep on top of, but stay healthy by keeping up with other activities, exercising regularly, eating well, and seeing friends and family.

CONCLUSION

While your elective rotations can be the most gratifying time of your medical school training, arranging them can be a fair amount of work and stress. You may start out with a well-thought-out strategy, but rarely will end up with a schedule that is exactly what you had planned. This is the case for everyone and particularly MD-PhD trainees who often face unique scheduling challenges during their training. By reading this book, you will understand that clerkship electives are just one of the steps on your career pathway toward becoming a physician-scientist. Ultimately, there are many ways of getting to the end (Chapter 27, "Career Choices After Graduation") and the training landscape is changing, which means you may need to forge your own way on this unique journey. So, take all advice about the strategic selection of your electives (including this!) with a grain of salt.

20

Integrating into a New Medical Class

Jiameng Xu

Jiameng Xu *is in the seventh year of the MD-PhD program at McGill University. She has recently completed her PhD in rehabilitation science. Her dissertation is an ethnographic study based in an inpatient psychiatry unit, which captures the lived experience of persons living with mental illness and their family members. Prior to entering medical school, she received a bachelor of science in life sciences, specializing in neuroscience, from Queen's University in Kingston, Ontario. She has also been involved in initiatives to create a space for the arts and humanities within health professional training and in spaces of health care delivery.*

INTRODUCTION

When I would tell my classmates that I was a student in the MD-PhD program and that I would be taking a leave of absence of 4 years to complete a PhD, I often received the response that I was being brave. I knew they were commending me for taking a leap. Yet a part of me believed I was not as brave as they imagined. The transition into clinical practice that they were imminently facing would begin for me in 4 years' time. In between, I would have the opportunity to learn something deeply important that would help me do the kind

WHAT YOU NEED TO KNOW

- Learning clinical medicine is a lifelong journey. The bumpiness of returning to medical school will pass.
- Ask for help. Everyone around you can be a teacher. Allow yourself to ask your classmates for an orientation, for example, or let your supervisors know if there is something in particular you want to practice or learn more about.
- Offer help. Reach out to other classmates who are returning to medical school after a leave of absence. Offer ideas and suggestions to those around you who are entering the world of research.
- Celebrate the strengths gained during your PhD studies. Do not be afraid to draw upon the learning and experiences you have gained during your graduate studies when it is pertinent to a clinical situation. Often, your classmates and colleagues will want to know about your research and what you have gained from it.
- Begin to work out your own ways of having a foot in both the worlds of clinical medicine and research. Give yourself time and curiosity to adjust to the culture of clinical medicine while holding on to the sensibilities you have honed while doing research.

of work I envisioned and that I believed would help me take better care of patients. In truth, I felt very fortunate to be able to return to medicine, that a space was being kept for me upon my return, and that I would still be allowed to reenter the class. I felt the security of someone who was going forth on a journey and had received the gift of a two-way ticket.

Elsewhere in this book, other authors dealt with essential adjustments of resuming medical training, such as transitioning to the wards (Chapter 18), selecting electives strategically (Chapter 19), standardized testing (Chapter 21), and preparing for residency applications (Chapter 22). I write this chapter to address the experiential aspects of returning to medicine and forming new relationships when joining a new medical class. Returning after a prolonged immersion in research is full of adjustments, calling for shifts in presence, perspective, and attitude. I wish to also address some of the worries, fears, and insecurities that might surround this transition, as well as the opportunities for growth in perspective contained in these challenges. Within the structure of the MD-PhD program, the proximity of research to the clinical world and one's first patient encounters with practicing medicine lay the groundwork for the creativity, translation, and bridge-building that will enrich clinical and research experiences thereafter. This chapter is about the formation of a new identity and about forming new relationships with one's colleagues and work.

PREPARING TO RETURN: PRACTICAL MATTERS

In the 12 months leading up to the return to medical school, there are a number of practical tasks that might require your attention. These administrative, financial, and logistical considerations were identified by Shira Ziegler in Chapter 18. Upper-year MD-PhD students, the undergraduate medicine education office, and medical classmates are resources that can help to guide you in preparing to return. Do not hesitate to ask questions and to reach out.

Two important considerations merit attention at the outset. One is to set up a plan for what portion of your PhD work, if any, will continue as you transition to the medical curriculum. That is, they submit their theses by the time they graduate from medical school, and defend their theses during residency. Although there are time pressures, it is important to give yourself the time that you need and to have a conversation with your PhD advisor and supervisory committee about this well in advance. The second key consideration is that the daily schedule in medical school will be less flexible compared to that of graduate studies. Matters that are more feasible to schedule during the PhD years, such as dental appointments, can suddenly become a challenge in medical school, sometimes requiring several weeks of approval for a half-day's leave of absence from clinical duties. It is a good idea to complete these tasks during the PhD if possible.

FACING IMPOSTOR SYNDROME

One of the greatest insecurities I had upon returning to medical school was how much I had forgotten. I remember the first time seeing a patient alone to conduct a physical exam, and my own hands faltering as I raised them over the patient's shoulders to palpate for the thyroid. The stethoscope felt like an unfamiliar object. Returning to medical school was akin to reacquiring a language I had forgotten. Sometimes, when the loss of confidence felt particularly acute, I had the sense that I was somehow less of a medical student. I remember thinking: *People look at me and think I am a third-year clerk, but they do not know that I have been away for 4 years.* During the time I have been doing research, medicine had also moved on—some of the guidelines and disease categorizations I seemed to recall had changed. Coming back was not as simple as picking up where I left off.

As time passed, I recognized another phenomenon I had not anticipated. As much as I focused on what I had difficulty recalling, I was also responding to everything I was learning through the lens of inquiry. I had decided to enter PhD studies to ask some fundamental questions. Now my questions had multiplied, and I was unable to take many things for granted, as I had done before. *Why does it work this way? Is this the optimal manner of doing things? Can this be otherwise? Where did this approach come from? Is there a pattern that cuts across situations? How does this relate to other things I have just learned?* Questions arose at every clinical encounter. I could not resist jotting down these questions and making field notes, as I had done during my PhD and clerkship. Being in the clinical environment stimulated questions I might have taken up as a PhD student and that I recorded after the clinical day was over.

I had heard several physician-scientists speak of the difference in culture between the world of clinical medicine and the world of research. Some of the differences were drawn at the pace, scope, and impact of the work. I was struck, however, by differences in emphasis and communication. In the first few months of clerkship, I realized that I was inclined to first present the pertinent negatives. Later, I realized that I had been carrying the mode of reasoning, in research, to reject hypotheses and to give due weight to negative data. This is used in clinical reasoning when ruling in and ruling out possibilities, but during communication, the positive findings needed to take precedence in order for an actionable clinical plan to be made. I was carrying ways of doing, knowing, and communication gained from the research world. Sometimes they aligned with those of the clinical world, and other times they differed.

A FOOT IN BOTH WORLDS

I learned that not only did I have to make room for new information and new ways of reasoning, looking at problems, and communicating my ideas, I needed to acknowledge that I already had a well-developed system of approaching problems and learning new things gained during my PhD studies. Whatever I learned anew in clinical medicine was going to be inevitably influenced by this system. I had to begin learning how they connect with one another.

Your perspective is valuable, and all the knowledge that you bring is to be celebrated

In classes on the role of the physician, we are advised to never underestimate the value of what we bring to the clinical encounter. We are told that our capacity to listen and be present to patients and their suffering form a powerful foundation to healing. The same can be said of the knowledge one already has, including research experience, brought to the clinical setting. I have heard the experience of starting each stage of clinical medicine described as starting once more at the bottom of the ladder. This holds some truth about the apprehension of approaching something that is completely new, to have to let go of previous security in one's knowledge and role. But this metaphor can be limiting and does not capture the possibilities of what you can bring to your clinical team and the clinical encounter. Every team I have joined is always at its capacity, and anything that students can contribute—an idea, a question, or other act of engagement—is helpful. Paul Savage, a contributing author in this book, advises a student approach every rotation with the mindset that it would be the field in which you would practice the rest of your career. My classmates, colleagues, and supervisors showed me that I could trust them to teach me well, as though I would be joining their profession or working with them for the long-term. The people around me made me that I was accepted. I was there to learn and to help.

Ask for help and accept offers of help

Returning to medical school can be disorienting. Sometimes the seemingly basic things, like how to access a curriculum database, can present a challenge. However, you will not be the only stranger, because clinical teams encompass more than just your peers. Introducing yourself to everyone, from the woman who sells you coffee in the morning to the unit coordinator to the residents and staff, will take you a long way to becoming integrated. Ask for help to navigate the new system you face. Importantly, you are likely to receive offers of help from classmates who recognize that a new student is joining their class after an extended leave of absence and who might not know anyone in the class at all. Accepting help can enable new friendships to grow. Asking for an informal orientation—about how information is communicated in the class, how students approach exams, study groups, or what clubs and interest groups are available—from others in the class can help you to settle in. Accepting help also meant accepting words of encouragement.

At the end of a unit, I described to my clinical supervisor my worries that I had forgotten too much and gotten mixed up about what appeared to be the fundamental facts. He assured me that I was actually at the level I needed to be. "Not knowing things applies to everyone," said a resident when I stated that I worried about my lack of knowledge. "We're all here to learn." Another clinician observed kindly, "At every stage of our training we feel like we are learning everything all over again. Third-year clerkship is its own learning stage, and fourth-year clerkship is its own, and residency after that, and entering your own practice." My classmates' and colleagues' responses showed me that the feeling of not knowing was common to everyone. This is also the time to not know, and to share your goals for your learning with your preceptors. Talk to your senior MD-PhD colleagues, who have also gone through this transition, and they will reassure you that though they also found this time to be challenging, no one expects you to have all the answers, and you will gain a sense of confidence with time.

Offer your knowledge; ask what your experiences and knowledge can contribute

We are often surrounded by colleagues who are entering the world of research for the first time, who have a question or clinical need they would like to address, or who are involved in a study. Sometimes, having a simple conversation about the Institutional Review Board process, or suggesting an online self-learning module, statistical toolkit, or someone whom they could speak to can help someone else progress in their research, and it is greatly appreciated. Others whom you meet in the clinical setting might need to learn the methodology you have used. Or you might become inspired by a clinical need to devise a research question and study around it. Another possibility is to connect with other students who are returning from a leave of absence for myriad reasons and to support one another in becoming oriented and navigating a new program. Never underestimate that you might be able to offer a suggestion that can help others around you navigate the research world and find their way to their own research collaborators, mentors, and resources.

Continue to ask questions of yourself, your thinking, and your work

Upon returning to the clinical environment, you may find yourself viewing clinical situations through the additional lens of your research training. Allowing yourself to ask questions and continue to be inquisitive can not only advance the care of patients, but also help you to gain insight into how research can be translated into practice, and how practice can inform research and make it clinically relevant. Many have found it helpful to keep a log or journal of the patients they have seen, both to keep track of their own learning and as a reference to later follow up on the outcomes for these patients and the clinical plans that had been acted on. It would also be useful to log moments that have surprised you. How might your research colleagues approach this issue? Are there gaps between the clinical and research perspectives? What would you wish for your colleagues to consider, for future medical and graduate students to be taught, for patients to be aware of? What are the priorities of clinicians, patients, and family members that are perhaps not being captured by the corresponding research area? What important element of clinical practice might the research community be missing? Is there an important clinical outcome that can be improved? Is there anything that might puzzle or even bother you about current practice? Do aspects of your participation in patient care call for certain questions to be raised and studied? Keeping a log of the research-related questions and ideas that arise during your transition back to medical school can be helpful for your later work. It is also important to not overextend yourself or feel guilty if you do not continue research during your return to medical school. Just as you have given research the dedicated time it deserved during your PhD, it is also appropriate if you feel you must do the same for your clinical training. Upper-year classmates have advised the importance of leaving time for self-discovery during clerkship and have highlighted there are many opportunities to pursue research later in residency.

A SENSE OF BELONGING

Whether we have spent some time away from medical school or not, we are all excited and apprehensive to enter the world of clinical medicine, where we are closer to patients and tangible action is taken. We can learn from each other's paths. Along every part of the journey, there are people who are farther ahead and show us that the way is possible. Gradually, I felt a sense of belonging grow. Although with every change of rotation, I would work with a new team of classmates, clinical colleagues, and supervisors, the familiar faces began to increase in number. Sometimes, on my way through the hospital to do a consultation, or in the cafeteria, I would stop for a minute to say hello or simply to wave across a distance. These familiar faces offered much comfort. Belonging came not only from becoming more used to the rhythms of work, which given the structure of clinical rotations eventually became the expectation to begin from a position of not-knowing, but also from the realization that every interaction turns a stranger into a colleague, acquaintance, and often a friend. It increased in seeing my classmates who were now senior residents or even practicing as general practitioners. If they made it that far, we would, too.

As time passed, the way I saw myself and my role also changed. Some of the initial feelings of being an impostor recurred. They were particularly strong whenever a new rotation began, but eventually time they held less power. My experience of clinical medicine, of being a learner, and of being part of a clinical team was no longer overshadowed by the acute awareness of being new and having been trained in a different domain. I came to see my place in terms of my own actions and the trust others placed in me. I started to see that in my role, the physical exam findings and history I had gathered helped the team come up with a clinical impression. The case report I wrote helped the inpatient unit better understand the multiple issues of a newly admitted patient. My attempts to translate a new diagnosis into lay terms helped a patient and family member better understand how to manage their condition at home and how to avoid having to come back to hospital. With each rotation, the language

I was speaking also changed rapidly. During team sign-overs, for example, when presenting a patient case at service rounds or communicating with a consultant, I realized that I was able to speak the language of medicine more fluently and less self-consciously than before.

Significant moments began to accumulate, drawing upon sensibilities and knowledge gained from both my PhD studies and from the clinical world. The sensibilities that my time during the PhD had instilled in me, which I had feared would be cumbersome or obstruct my view to what I would learn clinically, eventually found their purpose. They led me to bring articles to give to a patient who was interested in literature on her medication and its absorption post-bariatric surgery, articles that later held the interest of my clinical supervisor, who wished to have a copy for her own records. It was difficult to feel like an impostor when accompanying a patient through their dying process. Such intrusive thoughts did not appear when I found myself conducting the kind of narrative and phenomenological interview I had done during my ethnographic study, this time with an elderly patient to better understand her fears and desires with respect to receiving life-saving surgery. I still felt at times that my knowledge was wobbly, and faint traces of facts and terms remembered would often bump up against knowledge newly learned, but this slowly turned into something delightful and humbling, as though discovering that one can relearn how to ride a bicycle or to speak a language one might have forgotten with a deeper understanding and greater appreciation than the first time. I realized that much of my feeling of being an impostor stemmed from subconsciously comparing my reentrance into medical school with the major events that had immediately preceded it—the completion of PhD studies and the successful defense of my thesis, a rite of passage that was supposed to mark someone as being able to know. Recently, when I was called "doctor" by a patient and family member, I felt the familiar sense of embarrassment, but I no longer felt that I was pretending. I understood then a shift in my perspective. I was a true medical student and a true member of the team because I was doing my best to care.

CONCLUSION: TOWARD A PHYSICIAN-RESEARCHER PRAXIS

The time of transitioning back to medicine from research is a time to be treasured as an opportunity to live in the intersection of research and clinical practice. As much as the outward work of passing milestones is necessary, there is the less visible but equally important process of making clinical action a touchstone for inquiry, and vice versa. This integration can begin upon one's return to medical school and continues throughout residency, fellowship, or postdoc. It can manifest in seemingly mundane actions, such as practicing saying to our clinical colleagues what research we have done, or in more structured activities provided by our clinical environment, such as participating in service rounds and journal clubs. It is about the continuous formation of identity: finding your role as a physician-researcher, whatever that means for you. We also have the opportunity to facilitate meetings and relationships that might not otherwise happen. We can be a bridge, an interpreter, and a translator, bringing research relationships into the world of medicine, and clinical colleagues and even patients and family members into the world of research. Returning to clinical medicine is the beginning of seeing how the integration of knowledge creation and application can happen in the context of new relationships and new roles that will continue for a lifetime.

21

Standardized Testing—The USMLE and the MCCQE

Sarah Maritan • Joan Miguel Romero • Owen Chen

Sarah Maritan *is a first-year student in McGill University's MD-PhD program. She received her bachelor of science degree in life sciences and her master of science degree in pathology and molecular medicine, both from Queen's University. Her research focuses on the cellular signaling mechanisms regulating cancer progression, particularly the pathways underlying tumor cell movement and metastatic growth.*

Joan Miguel Romero *is a first-year MD-PhD student at McGill University. He completed his honors bachelor of science degree in pathobiology and immunology and his master of science degree in laboratory medicine and pathobiology from the University of Toronto. His research is aimed at understanding the antitumor immune mechanisms involved in pancreatic cancer.*

Owen Chen *is a first-year MD-PhD student at McGill University. Prior to medical school, he completed both his bachelor of science and master of science in biochemistry at McGill. He is currently pursuing his research at McGill's Rosalind & Morris Goodman Cancer Research Centre, where he studies cell cycle dysregulation in cancer.*

WHAT YOU NEED TO KNOW

- The United States Medical Licensing Exam (USMLE) is a three-part exam administered by the Federation of State Medical Boards (FSMB) and National Board of Medical Examiners (NBME); it is necessary for medical licensing in the United States.
- The Medical Council of Canada Qualifying Examination (MCCQE) is a two-part exam administered by the Medical Council of Canada (MCC), and it is part of the requirements to obtain a license to practice medicine in Canada.
- Various study resources exist for both tests, each with their own benefits.
- Deciding which to use is a matter of personal preference.
- Reasons for completing the USMLE and MCCQE exams differ depending on your career goals, and careful planning should determine which to take.

INTRODUCTION

In this chapter, we will discuss the USMLE and the MCCQE, exams necessary for becoming licensed to practice medicine in the United States and Canada, respectively. We will provide a basic rundown of what these exams are and why you would be interested in taking them. We then conclude with some study material that you may find useful.

UNITED STATES MEDICAL LICENSING EXAMINATION (USMLE)

What is the USMLE?

The USMLE is a standardized examination that is required for medical licensing in the United States, administered jointly by the Federation of State Medical Boards (FSMB) and the National Board of Medical Examiners (NBME). The USMLE consists of three steps: Step 1, Step 2, and Step 3. These are completed over multiple years during the course of your medical training. Specific timeline requirements to complete all three steps of the USMLE, particularly with respect to students in combined MD-PhD programs, can be consulted from the USMLE official website.

Step 1 is a multiple-choice computerized test that assesses your ability to apply basic science knowledge to clinical scenarios. Step 1 is traditionally taken during medical school, often between the preclinical years and the clinical rotations in the later years. Starting in 2022, the USMLE Step 1 will no longer be scored, but will instead be graded as pass/fail. No changes are currently expected for the USMLE Step 2 and Step 3 exams.

Step 2 is divided into two parts, Step 2 Clinical Knowledge (CK) and Step 2 Clinical Skills (CS), and both parts are usually taken between the clinical third and fourth years of medical school. Like Step 1, Step 2 CK is a multiple-choice computerized exam, but is more focused on the clinical science necessary for patient care, while Step 2 CS is a standardized patient encounter designed to evaluate patient-centered skills, including spoken English proficiency and communication, ability to demonstrate empathy, taking the patient's history, conducting the physical examination, and efficiency in writing a patient note. Step 2 CK results are reported as numerical scores, while Step 2 CS is assessed as pass/fail.

Step 3 is the final component of the USMLE and is completed during your residency program, commonly in the first 2 years. Step 3 is also a computerized examination where results are reported as numerical scores. However, unlike Step 1 and Step 2 CK, Step 3 spans over the course of two days and includes interactive cases. Step 3 is designed to assess your ability to manage a patient in a clinical scenario, including interpreting physical examination findings, ordering laboratory tests, and selecting treatment plans.

Why should you take the USMLE?

As discussed above, the USMLE is a series of exams necessary for practicing medicine in the United States as a licensed physician. It also plays an important role for applying to an accredited residency program in the United States. For Canadian medical students, the USMLE is optional, and taking it may be dependent on whether you'd like to register for an American residency or fellowship program after completion of your residency.

Broadly speaking, there are three categories of students who take the USMLE: (1) American medical school students or graduates who wish to pursue a residency program in the United States, (2) Canadian medical school students or graduates who wish to pursue a residency program in the United States, and (3) Canadian medical school students or graduates who wish to pursue a fellowship program in the United States. Some eligible medical students or graduates outside of Canada or the United States may also wish to attend either a residency or fellowship program in the United States. As this book focuses primarily on Canadian and American medical students, we focus on the three former categories.

1. Applying to an American residency program as an American medical student

In order to continue your medical training in the United States, you must enroll in an Accreditation Council for Graduate Medical Education (ACGME) accredited residency program. At most medical schools, the USMLE Step 1 is completed between second and third year; however, the exact timing will vary by institution. As mentioned above, completing Step 1 is required for applying to residency programs. Step 2 is also important, depending on your particular case and goals. It is worth mentioning that you will need to consider how your PhD studies may factor into your USMLE preparation schedule. The programs you are applying to, your specific situation, and timelines related to residency application must be taken into account when considering which step of the USMLE needs to be completed and at what time. Step 3 is not required, as this is completed during postgraduate training.

2. Applying to an American residency program as a Canadian medical student

As indicated, the USMLE is an exam for American medical students for advancement of their training and licensure. This is not the case for medical students in Canada, and completing or not completing the USMLE has no bearing on your training and licensing in Canada. However, you may decide to take Step 1 if you are planning to complete residency in the United States. As outlined above, you must consider how to schedule and optimize your studying for this exam, as this may be influenced by your PhD studies. Questions about Step 2, including requirements and timelines, can be addressed by your program of choice. It is also worth considering whether you apply to both American and Canadian residency programs since it may, at the time of writing this guide, indirectly affect eligibility to match to an American residency program. Further information can be found at the Canadian Residency Matching Service (CaRMS) official website.

3. Applying to an American fellowship program as a Canadian medical resident

You may also wish to complete residency training in Canada, followed by fellowship training in the United States. In this case, taking the USMLE may be required, depending on the fellowship program and whether you are interested in working secondary to your primary job as a fellow. Note that certain programs may also accept the MCCQE Part I and Part II (discussed below), as Canadian equivalents of the USMLE. To determine whether your fellowship of interest requires the USMLE and if so, which step of the USMLE, it is best to check with your program of choice.

Finally, given that completion of an American fellowship represents a career move well over 5 years in advance, deciding to completing the USMLE for fellowship requires dedicated planning, and you are advised to regularly check with the program for requirements, as these may change during the time you complete your PhD, clerkship, and residency training.

HOW SHOULD YOU PREPARE FOR THE USMLE?

Medical schools in the United States often incorporate USMLE preparation into their curriculum, so students have ample time and resources to tackle these grueling but important exams. In addition, some US medical schools hold in-class information sessions for registration and the exam application process. A few schools also have designated academic staff that meet with students regularly to check in on study progress. As discussed above, most US medical schools with 4-year programs recommend that students take Step 1 at the end of second year and Step 2 (CK and CS) between third and fourth year. Step 3 is taken during residency. Because Step 1 has typically been considered the hardest of the three steps, we will focus on preparing for Step 1. Further resources for Steps 2 and 3 can be found to supplement your studying.

Preparation time will vary depending on your study habits and the school you attend. Students may take anywhere from two months to a year or more to prepare for Step 1. Many medical schools recommend that students start studying at the beginning of second year and continue to study part-time throughout the year, considering the workload from regular classes. Those who need more time may even start partway through first year. Students are also often given a break from classes for several weeks to over a month some time at the end of second year, during which they can study for the exam full-time. However, the scheduled study time varies between schools. Some schools may even hold regular mock exam sessions throughout the first 2 years as a part of their medical curriculum. As individual study needs and school curricula scheduling can differ greatly, be sure to check with your own school to become familiar with its study timeline and exam resources. It is also a good idea to check the USMLE website on how to register and schedule your exam, as well as for more resources for exam preparation and other updates.

Since the USMLE is not required to apply to residency programs or to become a practicing physician in Canada, USMLE preparation and study time are not allocated in Canadian medical school curricula. However, for the reasons already mentioned, you may be a Canadian medical student planning on taking the USMLE. As outlined above, Canadian students should follow a similar timeline compared to that used by their US peers when studying for Step 1: begin studying at the beginning of the second year. It would be ideal to take a few weeks during the summer vacation period to study full-time prior to taking the exam. As outlined above, regardless of why you would complete the USMLE, it is important to consider how your PhD will affect your studying and when you decide to take the exam.

Books and online resources

In addition to the resources provided by your medical school, you may want to invest in other study tools to maximize your scores. There is a plethora of third-party resources that you may purchase with additional fees to help you to better prepare for these exams. As mentioned in Chapter 4 ("Standardized Testing—The MCAT"), the types of books and online resources that you use will depend on your study needs. Each resource available in the market will vary slightly in terms of the topics included, as well as the breadth and depth at which they are covered. For example, you may want to purchase a condensed study guide to use as a quick reference for all the major concepts and systems covered in the medical curriculum. This can serve as a refresher if you are having difficulties recalling a particular fact or understanding a concept that you learned a while ago. Resources like these will give you a superficial-to-adequate understanding of a large breadth of the material that may be tested.

In addition to using concise study guides, you may want to acquire other resources that cover topics more in depth, especially if you are struggling or have struggled learning them in the past, or if you are just not very familiar with them. There are numerous books and online resources—some dedicated to USMLE preparation, some not—that give in-depth explanations on topics such as pathology, microbiology, immunology, and pharmacology, just to name a few. These will certainly provide you with more reinforcement in your learning and studying for the exams. You may find it easier·to cover more ground while using a mix of both condensed and in-depth study tools tailored to your needs.

Many students will often study best when they do practice questions and mock exams, because they will get a better feel for the real exam and of course, learn from their mistakes. There is certainly a handful of companies that offer question banks and practice USMLE exams, along with answer keys with explanations. The company that you may use will depend on cost, reputation, comprehensiveness in the study material, and perhaps personal preference. While most resemble the real USMLE questions, and are widely used and praised by many students, remember that they are third-party resources and are not endorsed by the makers of the USMLE. Therefore, it is best to use these resources (should you decide to) along with staying updated by checking the official USMLE website.

USMLE website resources

As just mentioned, it is important to stay informed on the testing formats and material (no matter which step you are preparing to take), procedures on applying, and test dates by checking the USMLE website regularly. You will also find official preparation tools for each of the steps, other recommended resources, and answers to frequently asked questions regarding the exams.

Many students say that Step 1 of the USMLE is one of the hardest exams that you will take in your professional career, if not the hardest. If preparing for the MCAT is a marathon, preparing for this exam is an ultra-marathon. There is just so much material to go over that cramming would almost certainly result in a failing grade. This is why it is extremely crucial to plan out a study schedule early in the year and check in with colleagues, teachers, or mentors to make sure that you are on track. Pace yourself with the volume of studying: Studying for two hours straight daily will have bigger gains than studying for five to six hours while being distracted. Also, beware of burnout—this can be very easy, especially when reviewing everything you learned in your pre-clerkship years. Make time for personal wellness such as exercise and spending time with friends and family.

MEDICAL COUNCIL OF CANADA QUALIFYING EXAMINATION (MCCQE)

What is the MCCQE?

The Medical Council of Canada Qualifying Examination (MCCQE) is a standardized, two-part examination administered by the Medical Council of Canada (MCC). The MCCQE is divided into two exams. Part I is a computer-based section testing clinical decision making based on the CanMEDS (Canadian Medical Education Directives for Specialists) roles and is typically taken at the completion of your undergraduate medical school training. Part II is a role-playing section testing your professional competencies during clinical interactions, completed during residency. It is important to note that this is a progressive exam, and Part II can only be taken following the successful completion of Part I. Both parts must be completed in order to fulfill one of the requirements of the Licentiate of the Medical Council of Canada (LMCC), a necessary step to obtain a license to practice medicine in Canada.

HOW SHOULD YOU PREPARE FOR THE MCCQE?

The MCCQE Part I is in some ways similar in objective and layout to the USMLE Step 2 CK. It is a full-day, multiple-choice exam and is focused on testing clinical concepts. Students usually take about a month or two to prepare for the USMLE Step 2 CK, so it is best to set aside a similar amount of time to prepare for the MCCQE Part I. The MCCQE Part II tests candidates in an OSCE (Objective Structured Clinical Examination) format, similar to the Step 2 CS. The MCC website provides extensive preparatory materials for Parts I and II. They offer great sample questions and instructional videos on how to approach the different types of questions on the exams. It is important to check the MCC website regularly for any updates, information on exam registration, and other recommended study resources.

CONCLUSION

In this chapter, we discussed two important exams that you must complete as requisites to obtain licensure to practice medicine in the United States or Canada. We gave an overview of what the exams are, who may need to take them, and study materials that can help you prepare for these exams. Additionally, it is important to acknowledge that the structure and content of these tests might change in the years following publication of this book. The general recommendations stated in this chapter should still apply and be useful to you, but the specific ways in which these recommendations are implemented may need to be modified with changes to these tests in mind. Regardless of which exam you choose to take, or if you even decide to take both, completion of the USMLE and MCCQE represents two important milestones in your medical career.

22

Choosing the Right Residency, Applying, and Interviewing

Tianwei Ellen Zhou • Andrew Karaba

Tianwei Ellen Zhou *graduated from McGill University's MD-PhD program and is now is a resident in ophthalmology at Université de Montréal. Her PhD research focused on retinopathy of prematurity, a blinding eye disease that affects many premature infants.*

Andrew Karaba *is a fellow in infectious diseases at Johns Hopkins University. He completed his MD and PhD at Northwestern University, where his thesis research focused on herpes simplex virus pathogenesis. Following completion of the Medical Scientist Training Program he completed a residency in internal medicine through the Osler Medical Training Program at The Johns Hopkins Hospital.*

INTRODUCTION

Residency is the one step between a medical student and a full-fledged physician. For some people, residency is also the time to grow their career and family. It is a period that demands hard work and long hours. Your choice of program, therefore, is incredibly important. This decision will shape you professionally and personally. This chapter lists a number of significant factors that should influence your choice; as you are reading, we encourage you to make a very honest pros-and-cons list for each factor. The chapter will operate under the assumption that you have decided on your preferred specialty, perhaps thanks to your learning experience in your rotations, as discussed in Chapter 19. Even so, by no means is this an easy choice, and you do not need to make it alone. We encourage you to consult friends, colleagues, family, and resources, including this one. The process of becoming an intern once you have been accepted is the topic of the next chapter.

WHAT YOU NEED TO KNOW

- Match your residency location based on your career plan and lifestyle.
- Mentorship and didactic teaching are important for residents.
- For your interviews, be prepared and practice!
- Collect good stories from your clerkship so that you can use them in the interview.
- Take advantage of pre- or post-interview socials.

CHOOSING YOUR RESIDENCY

Location

The location of your residency program directly impacts your lifestyle. Large North American cities like New York, San Francisco, Chicago, Montreal, or Toronto offer fun summer festivals, dynamic art scenes, professional sports, and good restaurants—great places to relax and recharge when you are not on call. But traffic and rush hours are inevitable. Housing can be expensive. And finding a parking spot (if you can even reasonably maintain a car) can easily turn into a treasure hunt. You might be able to get around with public transportation, but keep in mind that you are often working odd hours, so residents may need a car. If you have children or are planning to start a family, moving to an area with a good school system or affordable housing becomes relevant. Will your significant other have job opportunities in the city? Is the city close to relatives (perhaps particularly important if you have children)? Other aspects to consider include the weather, availability of parks and museums, proximity to outdoor activities, as well as other amenities that are important to you and your family.

Mentorship and residency community

As a resident, you are learning many news things: time management, basic knowledge in your specialty, and the hospital systems. Having a supportive program goes a long way. So consider the following:

Is the program director available to residents (i.e., can they offer timely advice)? Ask the residents specifically what they like and dislike about the program director and how often they meet. People expect different things from a program director, so asking if they like the director is generally not sufficient. Various issues can arise throughout residency, such as conflicts between colleagues, unresponsive staff, limited equipment availability, expensive parking, or not knowing how to start a research project. A good program director—someone experienced and resourceful—can either provide you with prompt advice and potential solutions or point you to the right person for further details.

Another factor to consider is the culture of the program, for example, whether it fosters collaboration and is supportive. Coresidents can make or break a good residency. You are working together day and night for several years, so having a collegial environment will make an arduous residency more fun. You should not hesitate to ask how residents interact with one another inside and outside the workplace. Pay attention to tone and collegiality during residents' conversations and your rotations and electives (Chapter 19) if you have the opportunity to work with residents in a program you are considering for residency.

Learning opportunities

Residency teaching comes from didactic lectures and clinical services. There are several things that can impact the quality of residency education: Are there well-organized and well-attended didactic lectures to prepare you for the licensing and board examinations? Is there sufficient supervision during clinical service? Do they offer simulation experience? Attending conferences is another important aspect of teaching. Conferences offer opportunities to showcase your research and provide a chance to see new trends in your fields. But not all programs provide the same opportunity to attend conferences. Factors that might impact the ability to attend conferences include the size of the program, additional funding for conferences, and the amount of elective time.

WHAT TO PREPARE FOR THE INTERVIEW

The number of individual interviews, the types of questions, and the length of the interview day will vary considerably from specialty to specialty and program to program. However, you should dress professionally (interview suit), and be prepared to discuss anything on your application. For MD-PhD graduates, it is likely that part of the interview will focus on potential research mentors or projects you might be interested in. Therefore, you should think about what type of research you might want to focus on during residency. The content and types of questions you will be asked are quite varied. Many programs do try to encourage their interviewers to ask a few standard questions, so you might get the same question more than once.

In Canada, residency interviews examine the CanMEDS roles, a framework that describes key characteristics in a competent physician. These traits include: medical expert, professional, communicator, collaborator, leader, health advocate, and scholar. Keep in mind that each question presented during your interview essentially surveys at least one of these seven traits.

Remember, as you are being interviewed by the programs, you are interviewing the programs as well. Just like speed-dating, everyone in that interview room is trying to look for a good match within a very short amount of time. A pro tip: many medical schools have a list of interview questions "inherited" from senior students. Get your hands on those lists! It is likely that the most common question you are asked will be: "Do you have any questions about our program?" To address this, you should come up with a list of 15–20 things you want to know about every program. They should be things you can't find on the website but will give you a good sense of what the program is really like. For example, you could ask how many residents stay for fellowships or junior faculty positions, which indicates how happy residents are at that institution, or what the interviewer's favorite aspect of the program is.

Before heading to your residency interviews, it is a good idea to know yourself and the programs. Consider the following:

Know yourself	Know the programs
• Why did you choose this specialty? • Why should we choose you? • Your strengths and weaknesses (prepare 2~3 examples for each). Identify gaps and elaborate on how you will improve in the future. • Know your CV well. Be prepared to elaborate on anything mentioned in your CV. Be able to tie your past experience to why you are a good fit for a certain program. • Prepare some stories from your clinical experiences to reflect on teamwork, compassion, conflict resolution, and ethics.	• How is the program? How is the location? • The program's history and atmosphere (read about their website; do some online research; talk to current and past residents). • Their strengths and weaknesses. • Their curriculum and didactic teaching schedule. • Prepare some questions to ask during pre-interview socials and the interviews.

Telling a story using the STAR-L model

While it is relatively straightforward to tell the interviewers about yourself, many students find it more challenging to tell a story about a difficult experience. Here are some examples:

- Describe a patient who made an inappropriate (e.g., racial, gender, age) comment toward you or others. How did you feel? How did you handle it?

- Describe a time when you had to deliver bad news. How did you approach this conversation? How did the patient react? How did you handle your patient's reaction?

- Describe a situation when you got in a conflict with a colleague.

- Tell me about a time you did not get along with a superior.

- Tell me about a time when you made a mistake.

One trick I learned from my seniors is to accumulate a few relevant examples during your training. Almost all of us have encountered an unhappy patient or a misunderstanding between team members. Jot down those experiences and reflect on your feelings, your handling of the situation, the outcome, and what you had learned. Often, there is more than one way to handle a given situation. I encourage you to discuss your approach with family and friends who may have more life experiences. It is a great opportunity to see how others handle the same problem and to refine your answers.

During the interviews, the STAR-L model is widely used - Situation, Tasks, Actions, Results, and Lessons Learned - to tell a story and show interviewers your chain of thoughts. The STAR-L model is useful because it divides a complex situation into smaller pieces in a logical manner, making the story easier for the audience to follow.

- *S—Situation: Give the context to the situation (who, what, when, where) and explain why it was challenging.* As a fourth-year medical student, I was in an ophthalmology outpatient clinic and examined a gentleman in his seventies for his age-related macular degeneration (AMD). His disease ran an aggressive course; the left eye had no vision and his right eye was deteriorating rapidly. The imaging results indicated that his right macula had been irreversibly damaged by AMD. As such, he lost functional vision bilaterally.

- *T—Tasks: Describe the tasks you had to accomplish. Identify the difficulty in the context of the situation.* Being an energetic person all his life, the patient had a true passion for golf. He had always feared that this hobby would be stripped away by the disease. Unfortunately, I had to inform him that not only he would not be able to play golf, but also he'd need help for daily living from this point forward.

- *A—Actions: What did you do? Describe how the story played out.* I sat down with the patient and his daughter. I succinctly recapped the course of his AMD management. I also mentioned that during the last two visits, the team had discussed the possible outcome (blindness) with the patient. With a slow and sympathetic tone, I told him that currently there is no treatment for AMD, but I could connect them to resources that helped patients adapt to a life with visual impairment. During our conversation, I paused regularly and encouraged both of them to ask questions.

- *R—Results: Describe how the situation played out, good or bad.* The patient was visibly discouraged. He was stone-faced and remained quiet most of the time. The disappointment was palpable. However, both the patient and his daughter asked several questions about the vision-impairment support groups and were motivated to be connected.

- *L—Lessons learned: State the lessons you learned from this scenario.* There are a few things to be learned in this case: (1) When revealing bad news, it is essential to take your time and recap the disease progression and its management with the patients. In doing so, patients have a better understanding of the natural history of this condition. They are more prepared to hear the final outcome. (2) The revelation of bad news should always be a conversation. Often, patients are already overwhelmed by emotions. So, I made use of small pauses, allowing them to clear their thoughts and ask questions.

Recycling your answers

We only have a limited number of stories, but there are endless ways for interviewers to ask questions. Hence it is important to recognize that some questions can be grouped together and learn to recycle your answers.

For example, the above mentioned "breaking bad news" example can be also used as a story for effective communication between a trainee and a patient, or for managing your emotion in an uneasy situation. Another example: you can address your weakness as doing too many things at the same time. The same issue could be mentioned in your time management skills: "At first I tried to jam too many research projects at the same time; but it turned out I was not able to finish the tasks on time. I gradually learned to politely decline additional projects and to focus on the current tasks. In doing so, I was able to close the loop on my research projects and publish these studies. I also learned the importance of prioritizing."

Practice, practice, practice!

Now that you have written down key points to your questions, the next step is to practice. This can be done with friends or family. Before interviews, Dr. Zhou got together with trusted friends from medical school. We knew each other well and were aware of each other's strengths and weaknesses. In addition, we agreed to share our opinions openly and discuss issues objectively. The upside to practicing with medical school friends is that all of us had gone through the same process and understood medical training well. The downside could be a lack of patients' perspectives. So, in addition to practice with classmates, I also practiced with family members. They provided me their viewpoints as patients and what they wished to hear from their doctors. Their stories about bad doctors were quite valuable, as I learned from the mistakes made by others. Alternatively, many medical schools will offer mock interviews with faculty at your current medical school to prepare for the real residency interviews.

Addressing a question for the first time is often the most difficult—you may tell too many or too few details of story; you may not be using the most appropriate words; you may forget to mention something important; or you may simply forget your lines. Prepare for the interview ahead of time, practice a few times before friends and family, and refine your answers before heading to the real thing.

What are appropriate and inappropriate questions?

Both the Accreditation Council for Graduate Medical Education (ACGME) and the Canadian Resident Matching Service (CaRMS) have clear guidelines about what subjects and types of questions are off-limits in an interview. Before interviewing, it would be wise to familiarize yourself with them.

Here are a few appropriate and inappropriate questions.

Appropriate to ask	Inappropriate to ask
• Gaps and absence in education. • What has your experience been in working with people in authority? • How do you learn best? • Are you legally entitled to work in Canada or the United States?	• Your personal life (e.g., marriage status, if you have or want children or not, etc.) • Where were you born? • How old are you? • What is your ethnic background? • What is your sexual orientation? • What is your religion? • What is your first language? • To what other programs did you apply? • Have you received other interviews? • Do you plan to rank our program?

TAKE ADVANTAGE OF THE PREINTERVIEW SOCIALS

Most programs organize a social or dinner the day before or after the interview. Details for the social are included in the invitation emails, so please go through those emails carefully.

These gatherings with drinks and food offer a great opportunity for candidates to get to know people in the department and to learn more about the program. How does the call schedule look? When do people know what subspecialty they'd like to pursue? Where do residents live? What do residents do for fun? These questions are appropriate for a professional discussion and a lighthearted chat. This is a critical way to gauge the camaraderie (or lack thereof) of a program.

It is always wise to be professional and polite during these gatherings. Drinking in moderation or not at all should be the basic consensus. Though it is hard to set candidates apart simply by preinterview socials, programs do red-flag candidates if they misbehaved, for example, if they were highly inebriated or uttered inappropriate comments. Interviews are often held during a condensed few months, and many interviews take place on consecutive days; therefore, careful planning is needed if you want to attend all the social events as well as interviews.

CONCLUSION

It is not easy to organize interviews for candidates from across the country. At the end of your interview, take a minute to thank the interviewers for this opportunity and the supporting staff for managing the logistics. After that, I encourage you to take 10–15 minutes in a quiet setting to reflect upon the good and not-so-good answers. First, were there anticipated (and hence well-prepared) questions? Second, were there questions that caught you off-guard? If so, why? One common technique to counteract this is to recycle your answers. Finally, write down the questions that surprised you and think about whether you answered them in the best way possible. If you didn't, what would have been a better answer? Importantly, do NOT be too hard on yourself for less-than-perfect answers. We tend to be more conscious (and more self-critical) of our perceived mistakes than other people are, and it is more constructive to learn from them.

Increasingly, the ACGME is limiting post-interview communication between candidates and programs. It used to be quite common for candidates to send thank-you notes to the program director and interviewers, but this is discouraged now. If you have lingering questions about the program that were not answered during the interview, then you should reach out to the program contact (usually the program director), but otherwise you should not contact the program. No post-interview contact is becoming the norm. If and when you are accepted, congratulations! It's time to move on to the next step of your journey: becoming an intern (Chapter 23).

Part V

Residency, Fellowship, and Your First Job

23

Becoming an Intern

Shira G. Ziegler

Shira G. Ziegler *graduated from The Johns Hopkins University School of Medicine MD-PhD program in 2018. Her graduate research elucidated the mechanisms underlying rare disorders of ectopic calcification and identified potential treatment strategies. She is currently pursuing dual residency training in pediatrics and medical genetics at The Johns Hopkins Hospital and plans to combine her bench-to-bedside research on rare genetic conditions with clinical care. Prior to medical school, Shira graduated from Oberlin College with highest honors in neuroscience and worked in the National Institutes of Health's Undiagnosed Diseases Program and Human Genome Research Institute.*

INTRODUCTION

You walked across the stage, donned not one—but two!—academic hoods, and finally graduated with your MD and PhD degrees. You did it! While you can revel in being called double doctor from mid-May to mid-June, you soon will be thrown into intern year along with several other newly minted physicians. Your choice of residency (Chapter 22), significant as it was, was just the prelude to this stage. Intern year is the first year of residency and your first year as a practicing doctor. It is challenging, filled with steep learning curves and tireless call schedules. Also, while you have just spent the last 7–10 years training to become a physician-scientist, for most internships, your year will be solely focused on clinical training. You will have to hang up your lab coat and sport your white coat (or embroidered fleece) and spend most of your time in the emergency departments, wards, intensive care units, and operating rooms.

YOU'RE NOT ALONE

While intern year is highly variable depending on the selected specialty, there are shared experiences. Intern year is fundamentally about learning the difference between sick and not sick. You will be entrusted to be the first call for your patients. You will be the first to

---

WHAT YOU NEED TO KNOW

- As an intern, your purpose is no longer to impress your peers.
- Learn how to safely, efficiently, and empathetically treat patients.
- Create a support network of friends, family, colleagues, and hospital resources.
- Take advantage of dedicated rest time granted by an inflexible schedule.
- Consider the research tracks and physician-scientist training programs at your institution of choice.

their bedside and the first person to answer questions, talk to family members, and dictate care plans. While novel and exciting, it can also be intimidating and harrowing. You will be confronted with life-altering, critical decisions, and sometimes death. Lean on your co-interns and learn from your senior residents and attending physicians. Remember that you can ask for help. No longer are you a medical student trying to impress your teams and be self-sufficient. You are a doctor, and your sole purpose is to learn how to safely, efficiently, thoughtfully, and empathetically diagnose and treat patients.

Intern year can also provoke feelings of inadequacy, frustration, and fatigue. Try to make time to process these feelings and recognize burnout. Participate in the extracurricular activities that you enjoyed during medical and graduate school. Read, draw, run, hike, cook. Find the time to do something that you love. Create a support network of family and friends. Also, essentially all hospitals have mental health and wellness resources. Identify and seek out those resources. If you are having trouble accessing these services, talk to your program leadership or residency director. Schedule annual physical exams and biannual dentist appointments. Remember to also take care of *your* physical health.

SCHEDULING FOR A MANAGEABLE WORKLOAD

During intern year and throughout residency, your schedule will be predetermined. While the inflexibility is jarring compared to your graduate school days, take advantage of having a dedicated one to two weeks of vacation twice a year without research or clinical responsibilities. Whether it is a staycation or international travel, make sure to protect the time and use it for a reprieve from the hours spent taking care of others.

On a practical note, if possible, try to outsource tasks. Many interns and residents pay for dog walkers, house cleaners, car washers, grocery shoppers, and food delivery services. Also, try to take the United States Medical Licensing Exam (USMLE, addressed in Chapter 21) Step 3 early in your training, preferably during intern year. Step 3 content is very similar to Step 2 and includes a breadth of topics and clinical scenarios such as medicine, pediatrics, women's health, and surgery. It is much easier to study for the exam earlier on in your training, while the Step 2 content is still fresh, before you dive into your chosen specialty. It is usually recommended to study for Step 3 for two to four weeks during a clinical block with a lighter workload. Make sure to coordinate with your chief residents before obtaining your scheduling permit and committing to an exam date to ensure your availability.

CONTINUING YOUR PHYSICIAN TRAINING

Many academic institutions have research tracks and physician-scientist training programs. Physician-scientist training programs are aimed mainly at residents and fellows in their research years to provide resources such as grant-writing workshops and fellowship application opportunities. As you transition out of intern year and into years with opportunities for research electives, consider getting involved. Refer to Chapter 24 for more information on how to pursue research during residency training.

CONCLUSION

Overall, throughout intern year, try to maintain perspective. While this might just be another day for you in the hospital, or hour 26 of a 28-hour shift, remember that for your patients, this is likely their worst day and possibly their worst hour. Intern year will provide the foundation for the rest of your clinical training and hone your clinical skills. Take advantage of this opportunity and recognize the privilege.

24

Integrating Research into Residency

R.J. Doonan

R.J. Doonan *is a fourth-year vascular surgery resident at McGill University. He completed his MD-PhD at McGill University, investigating new methods to identify unstable carotid plaques through clinical, translational, and basic science approaches. Throughout residency, he has also pursued outcome research in aortic aneurysm treatment and advanced endovascular therapies for complex abdominal and thoraco-abdominal aortic aneurysms. When not working, R.J. enjoys cycling, hiking, and spending time with his partner Pauline and his two dogs Ellie and Oliver.*

INTRODUCTION

Conducting and completing a high-quality research project is an extremely rewarding experience, and this remains true during residency. It is entirely possible to succeed in residency both academically and clinically. The long hours, significant clinical responsibilities, and pressure to continue to produce good research will prove difficult but surmountable. This chapter will provide insight into what to expect when trying to integrate research into residency, tips and tricks to help you succeed, types of research to conduct during residency, and work-life balance.

Different people enrolled in different programs in places around the world will have varying experiences. While some of what I will tell you here is an amalgamation of other residents' experiences, advice, and observations, much of this chapter is based on my own experience. Be aware of that bias. Not everything will apply directly to your unique situation. I suggest taking everything written here into context and with a healthy dose of skepticism.

WHAT YOU NEED TO KNOW

- Develop short- and long-term goals and objectives. Discuss them with others. Check your progress and reassess them regularly.
- Build upon your foundational skills but take the time to learn something new.
- Find at least one mentor who can help guide you through your physician-scientist development.
- Setting realistic expectations for research commitments before starting residency will shape your experience in a positive way.
- Your own well-being should be your number one priority. Take care of yourself and seek help if needed.

TIPS AND TRICKS FOR SUCCESSFUL RESEARCH INTEGRATION IN RESIDENCY

Set goals/objectives

Similar to the goals and objectives of each of your individual rotations, setting research goals and objectives is important in preparing for success. I suggest setting short- and long-term goals, which may translate into yearly and residency-long goals. These goals can guide you from your intern year, as discussed in Chapter 23, until you secure your first job, the topic of Chapter 26, and beyond. They could encourage engaging in a particular number of research projects, publications or conference presentations, learning new skills, awards and grants, research fellowships, and more. This exercise will help you stay focused throughout the year and direct your efforts. You may have several research project possibilities, but which one aligns most with your own objectives? Making decisions becomes much easier when you have clear, guiding goals. Those goals should be reasonable and reevaluated frequently. If you are very far from achieving a specific objective, is it because it's too lofty or because you need to apply yourself better? What are the barriers to your success? Taking time to reflect on these issues, and others will help you stay on track.

Going forward, most of your career, clinical, and research objectives will be linked. During residency (and fellowship), your clinical and research interests may become more closely related than during your MD-PhD training, as you slowly develop an area of interest as a practicing physician-scientist. As you progress through your training, at least some of your goals and objectives should become more focused to set you up for fellowships and/or securing a physician-scientist position.

Some examples of my own goals and objectives included:

Post-Graduate Year 1
- Focus on being a good physician and junior resident.
- Develop groundwork for research projects for the following year (this goal changed from the original "start one longitudinal project and two to three cross-sectional projects early in year one of residency," which was too ambitious).

Post-Graduate Year 2
- Improve sewing skills and groin dissections.
- Improve medical student teaching.
- Conduct, complete, present, and publish one research project.

Post-Graduate Year 3
- Lay appropriate groundwork for aortic pathology research projects to be presented and published during fourth year.
- Transition to increased independence in the operating room.

Post-Graduate Year 4
- Increase my visibility within the vascular surgery community, specifically within the aortic community.
- Publish three manuscripts on aortic pathologies, including advanced endovascular treatment of complex aortic aneurysms.
- Present at four conferences, including at least one specialized aortic conference.
- Secure advanced open and endovascular aortic fellowship training.

It is clear that my examples are varied. However, you will notice they include objectives for different aspects of my physician-scientist career development. This list was also made while keeping the goals of past and future years in mind. In third year, I set myself up for research projects that would allow me to increase my visibility within my surgical community, with the goal of securing additional training to become a vascular surgeon with a specialized interest in aortic surgery. Succeeding at my R4 goals was enabled by the successful completion of my R3 goals. There were, of course, many more objectives than shown here, and these were in flux throughout my training. Most important is that once you have a list of objectives, develop a plan to obtain these goals and execute your plan.

Develop a plan and stress-test it

Next you need methods with which you will achieve these goals. Simple and specific goals such as publishing a manuscript may be relatively easy to achieve. Goals that are broader, particularly ones that involve career direction or the intersection of clinical and research objectives, require significant planning.

Before developing an approach for each objective, it is important to recognize barriers to successfully achieving each goal. These may not be obvious, so I suggest discussing your goals with colleagues and your mentor(s). They will help gauge the difficulty and approach that may be best. It will also be an opportunity to help determine if your specific objectives will actually help direct you toward your broader long-term goals. Ultimately, developing a good plan and identifying obstacles will allow you to be flexible in your methods while never losing sight of your goals.

Build upon the skills developed during your MD-PhD

There is no doubt that you came out of your MD-PhD training a different person than when you entered. Your knowledge and abilities likely increased dramatically, and there are several skills you learned that could be directly applicable to some of the research you will conduct during residency. Use these well-developed skills, and continue to refine them. For example, if you gained significant experience in statistical analysis of large data sets during your PhD, seek out a project where this skill can be applied. Your skills will be an asset to the project, you will be able to complete the work in significantly less time compared to during your PhD, and you will likely obtain a publication from this investment.

Try something new

As part of your academic career development, it is also crucial to try new things and acquire new skills. If your situation allows you to either work in the same field as your PhD or even with the same principal investigator, try to branch out. This does not mean to cut ties and change direction completely, particularly if you are passionate about your current area of interest. However, at least a portion of your time should be dedicated to exploring new avenues of research with different people in different fields and learning new things. This will enrich your professional development and ultimately refine your physician-scientist toolbox.

Engage with other residents/medical students

Working on a research project solo may be right for you. It may even be your preferred approach to conducting research. However, most good research cannot be performed alone. Therefore, it benefits you to learn early on how to work in a team.

There are many other benefits to working together with residents on a research project. First, you can split the workload to keep up with your research deadline. Second, you will learn from one another. Third, if you are working with a less-experienced resident, you will have an opportunity to mentor and teach a colleague. Mentoring students and residents will be a useful skill your whole life. Team research projects are an opportunity to practice.

Naturally, there is potential for conflict. Remember to elect the person with whom you will work carefully. Outlining roles and responsibilities, targets, and clear authorship and conference-presentation roles is paramount. The authorship agreement should be made before starting the project, and the discussion should include other coauthors, if applicable, and your research supervisor. Get the agreement in writing. An email summarizing your discussions should suffice. It is easiest if the work you are doing will lead to multiple publications. Then you can collect data together, each analyzing your own data, and write your own manuscripts with support from each other. Bottom line, clear communication before starting a project with a colleague will save you heartache later on. Chapter 13 ("Publication") included some more advice on the necessary cooperation that goes into creating publishable papers.

Find a mentor

The importance of having good mentorship cannot be understated. You should find at least one mentor who will help guide you in planning and achieving your goals and objectives. I also believe that as a physician-scientist, it is important to not only have a research mentor to help guide your research endeavors, but also someone to help navigate your clinical training and career development.

You may prefer to have more than one mentor. They can offer different perspectives and guidance in multiple areas. Your mentor(s) can be from your own department, outside your department or institution, a collaborator, or even someone assigned to you by a mentorship matching program. Key qualities of a mentor include a willingness to share their skills, knowledge, and expertise while guiding and motivating you in your own career development. Regardless of where or how you connect with your mentor, ensure that you share with them your thoughts and ideas on your own plans and objectives. Their input can be invaluable.

Time management and resource utilization

The most significant roadblock to research productivity during residency is likely time. It is important to manage your time efficiently and identify and utilize available resources within your division, department, or university. This includes strategic planning of research electives or protected research time. I suggest scheduling protected time to maximize completion of research tasks that are inflexible and cannot be executed part-time while performing clinical duties. Examples include multi-day benchwork experiments or direct collection of patient samples (more on types of research below). Upon return to clinical activities, you can then perform tasks that are more flexible, such as data analysis or manuscript preparation.

Many divisions (even small ones) have dedicated personnel such as research coordinators for divisional research support. Some may have dedicated tasks such as coordinating clinical trials, but still inquire about availability of research personnel for support on your projects, as well as any other resources, including divisional funding, statistical software, or access to previously developed data sets. It never hurts to inquire what support can be assigned to your own projects.

TYPES OF RESEARCH

Basic science

Most readers will come from a basic science background with strong willingness to continue. The upside to pursuing basic science research during residency is that you will be unique. Most residents will not perform basic science research, except for a small percentage of those who take time off for a master's or PhD. Basic science also allows you to delve deep into mechanisms of diseases you are now encountering on the wards, a true bench-to-bedside approach.

Basic science also comes with a significant downside. It is extremely time-consuming, relatively inflexible, and can often not be put on hold for several months during busy rotations. You will not be able to produce basic science research of significance during residency without a convergence of circumstances.

Using protected research time may be the simplest method to conduct basic science research during residency. Opportunities for long periods of research electives, fellowships, or post-doctoral training may be possible during residency at your institution. However, not all residency programs will support long periods of research time. If you wish to pursue this path, ensure your program will allow for the required time away from clinical duties, and plan far in advance, if possible.

Another possibility is for research coordinators, technicians, or associates to perform experiments on your behalf while you act as a junior principal investigator. This type of agreement with your principal investigator is rare. It may be possible if there is extra funding or if your principal investigator wants to further support your work. You can even write and submit an operating grant to fund your proposed project. This should be discussed with your principal investigator toward the end of your PhD, since funding will need to be available early during residency to carry out your work.

The least desirable option for conducting basic science research during residency is by having a colleague or research assistant conduct maintenance on your behalf (e.g., animals or cell lines), while you spend evenings and weekends performing experiments. I DO NOT recommend this option. It requires most of your free time be spent in the lab, to the detriment of clinical study time and physical and mental health. If you are performing the bulk of your experiments, in addition to full-time residency training, you will underperform in at least one area and put yourself at risk for burnout.

For most residents, basic science research without protected research time during residency is not the optimal choice unless you have extremely strong support that will prevent your clinical training from suffering.

Clinical and epidemiological research

For the majority of residents, clinical or epidemiological research is the clear choice. It typically involves analyzing data that is pre-collected or collecting clinical data that has been recorded elsewhere. This flexibility is crucial, and projects can be tailored to be short and simple, large and broad, or prospective. It also allows asking and answering research questions developed from current clinical experiences. This form of research may require a background or willingness to learn institutional requirements for patient-centered research, database management, and statistical analysis. Despite this, clinical and epidemiological research circumvents the cons of basic science and is likely the appropriate choice for balanced physician-scientist training during residency.

CHALLENGES OF INTEGRATING RESEARCH DURING RESIDENCY

Challenges of research integration during residency will be unique to each reader based on many factors, including research background and current and potential research activity within your residency program. However, there are some universal truths to integrating research during residency that I wish I knew beforehand:

First, performing good-quality research during residency while trying to become an excellent physician is difficult. It was certainly much harder than I expected. I had been able to start my PhD project in the early years of medical school, and my schedule and familiarity with the topics helped me to continue work on several projects while I completed my last years of medical school.

I began residency thinking I would start a longitudinal project and work on one or two easier cross-sectional projects to produce publications early in training. After the first few months, I found myself burdened by clinical responsibilities and expectations and the drive to be an excellent physician. After all, many non–physician-scientists believe that physician-scientist trainees make weaker physicians, especially in surgery. I had to prove them wrong. I found it very difficult to get started on research projects early in residency, and I felt I was being pulled in different directions.

This was all because my own expectations were clearly too ambitious. I encourage you set more reasonable expectations by developing appropriate goals and objectives, and discussing these with mentors and colleagues.

Second, as an MD-PhD graduate, you may be the person with the most research experience in your residency program. In fact, you may have more experience than some of your attendings. That makes you an asset to your program, and they will want to tap into your potential.

You will be highly sought after to participate in research projects. However, not all projects offered will be in your best interest. Evaluate every opportunity for what you and others will gain but also what opportunities could potentially be lost due to participation in a given project. Do not take this as a suggestion to be completely egocentric and only participate if there is a large upside for your career. Simply understand that not all opportunities will be of equal value, and your time is precious.

Third, clinical training will be physically and emotionally exhausting, with periods over an academic year that will be more or less productive in terms of research output. I often felt if I did not work on my research project for a few weeks that I was failing. I had not accepted the cyclical nature of research productivity that is sometimes required in order to similarly excel at one's clinical training. Compartmentalizing periods of time for primarily clinical work or primarily research was very useful and gave me improved focus.

Finally, an MD-PhD degree will be looked upon with vastly different opinions and judgments depending on the person and context. Remember that you pursued this combined degree to provide yourself with the training required to be in position to lead and advance your field. There will be doubters with a chip on their shoulder trying to compete for research prowess, just as there will be people who will look to you as a research authority figure. Be prepared to accept and manage these interactions.

WORK-LIFE BALANCE AND BURNOUT

Work-life balance can include personal interests, family, and social or leisurely activities. For many, this means spending quality time with friends or family, physical activity, reading, or playing an instrument. My own idea of work-life balance involves spending time with my partner and our two dogs. We love to explore new areas and hike. When I do not have time to leave the city to go hiking, I will take my dogs on a walk or play fetch in the park. They keep me grounded and are arguably the most important factor to my wellness. I also sometimes use my extra research commitments as opportunities for wellness. If a colleague and I are working on a Sunday morning on research, when we would otherwise have time off, I might recommend we work through the morning then grab lunch together outside the hospital.

I have many friends, colleagues, and mentors who are long-distance runners, avid cyclists, triathletes, or participate in ironman races. Whether you like to cook, bake, spend time with family, exercise, paint, or anything else, find something that you do regularly that takes you away from work. Make this activity a real priority. It should not be the first thing you stop doing when you get busy. Taking care of yourself can help avoid burnout.

Burnout is a syndrome manifesting as signs of physical, mental, and emotional exhaustion as a result of work-related stress. It includes feelings of depersonalization, loss of personal achievement, reduced performance or productivity, cynicism or negative attitude, fatigue, low mood, or difficulty concentrating. Burnout has become a critical issue in medicine only recently, and its importance has risen rapidly. In my own specialty, surgeons who met criteria for burnout are twice as likely to be depressed and to have suicidal ideation, underscoring its importance.

Unfortunately, trainees are not exempt and meet burnout criteria in similar proportions to physicians. Medical schools and residency programs have become more tuned in to the issue than in decades past. Significant time pressure, chaotic environments, low control of pace and environment, electronic medical records, and responsibility conflicts between home and work have all been identified as important causes of burnout.

A number of interventions have been shown to mitigate the risks of burnout, including a healthy work-life balance and adding flextime to physician schedules. But as residents, we have minimal control over our schedules and which electronic medical record systems our hospitals employ. We often live in chaos. Therefore, building your work-life balance and developing a support network are crucial.

However you decide to formulate your own work-life balance, please know that you are not immune to burnout. If you are experiencing burnout, you are certainly not alone. Reach out to your fellow residents regularly; they know what you're going through. Having a support system is key to preventing and mitigating burnout. If you have a partner, it is important that they are supportive and understanding. A partner who shares in responsibilities at home, as well as your successes and difficult times at work, will often be the most important part of your support network. Seek help from friends, colleagues, your program director, and resources from your university, residency, or specialty society. Your mental health is important to you and everyone around you, including your patients, family, and friends. The more we discuss these issues, the more likely we are to be able to identify and treat the root causes.

CONCLUSION

Integrating research into residency is an important part of continued physician-scientist career development. Ultimately, there is no magic formula for success in this endeavor, and it will require an individualized, deliberate approach. With proper motivation and direction, you can successfully integrate research into residency, publish high-impact manuscripts, and advance your field. Your continued effort during this time will pay dividends later.

25

Clinical Fellowship and Postdoctoral Training

Andrew Karaba

Andrew Karaba *is a fellow in infectious diseases at Johns Hopkins University. He completed his MD and PhD at Northwestern University, where his thesis research focused on herpes simplex virus pathogenesis. Following completion of the Medical Scientist Training Program, he finished a residency in internal medicine through the Osler Medicine Training Program at The Johns Hopkins Hospital.*

INTRODUCTION

After spending 10 or more years getting an MD, a PhD, and completing residency, you may feel you are finally ready to live the physician-scientist dream and start a lab while spending a portion of your time doing clinical work. However, many MD-PhDs complete one final step in their medical and scientific training before launching their career. This period of training is referred to as fellowship. Fellowship is a time to refine your clinical interests in a subspecialty (such as gastroenterology, pediatric nephrology, cardiac anesthesia, or dermatopathology) and sharpen your research skills before you are truly on your own. This chapter will describe fellowship, important considerations in choosing a fellowship for MD-PhDs, how to make the most of your fellowship, and briefly describe what comes next.

WHAT IS A FELLOWSHIP?

A fellowship is a period of training after residency that can last as little as 1 year and as long as 5 years depending on your specialty, the specific fellowship program, and your goals. Nearly all fields of medicine have subspecialties. Urogynecology is a subspecialty of

---

WHAT YOU NEED TO KNOW

- Fellowship provides subspecialty clinical training as well as research training.
- Most MD-PhDs complete a fellowship, but this is specialty-dependent and may not be necessary to have a career as a physician-scientist.
- Research might be combined with residency if you pursue a research pathway.
- Choosing a fellowship mentor is a critical decision.
- When choosing a fellowship program, select one whose graduates have the type of jobs you desire.

gynecology, rheumatology is a subspecialty of both internal medicine and pediatrics, and colorectal surgery is a subspecialty of general surgery. The list of all subspecialties is quite extensive. The purpose of the fellowship is twofold: to gain additional clinical skills necessary to be a subspecialist and to pursue scholarly activities. Most fellowships have both clinical and research periods to accomplish these goals. The clinical portion is similar to residency in that a fellow will see and treat patients under the supervision of a more senior attending physician. The research portion can take many forms. It can look very much like a traditional postdoctoral fellowship in which the fellow is working in the lab of a senior scientist (principal investigator or PI). However, some fellows pursue more clinically focused projects in which they spend their research time acquiring additional analytical skills in order to do clinical research under the guidance of their mentor. The process of applying to a fellowship begins in residency.

For example, if you want to become a cardiologist who treats adult patients, you would need to complete a residency in internal medicine, which is typically 3 years in the United States and Canada. During the third year of residency you would apply to cardiology fellowships, interview, create a rank list (like residency selection), and eventually match to a cardiology fellowship. Then you would spend at least 3 years learning how to be a clinical cardiologist and to conduct research related to cardiology. This process is similar for nearly all internal medicine and pediatric subspecialties (such as nephrology, pulmonology/critical care, infectious diseases, rheumatology, and oncology). However, many fellowships in surgical subspecialties are only 1 year long, do not have a formal matching process, and do not have dedicated research time built in. Some fellowships are accredited by the Accreditation Council for Graduate Medical Education (ACGME), which is the same body that regulates and oversees residency programs. These fellowships will have a similar structure at all institutions and are subject to duty-hour restrictions and other programing deemed necessary by the ACGME. Others are ACGME-equivalent, meaning they adhere to the same regulations but are not actually under ACGME jurisdiction, and some have nothing to do with the ACGME. The point is, the length of the fellowship, how time is allocated, and the application process vary from specialty to specialty. Much of what is described in this chapter is geared toward those fellowships that offer protected research time.

The dedicated clinical training during fellowship is often time-intensive, and it would be difficult to be very productive from a research perspective. During the protected research time, your clinical responsibilities are often minimal and may be only a half-day of outpatient clinic once per week or the occasional overnight call. The rest of the time is yours to pursue research.

DOES EVERY MD-PhD GRADUATE COMPLETE A FELLOWSHIP?

While the subspecialty clinical training and protected time for research are the primary reason to pursue a fellowship, not every MD-PhD needs to (or should) complete one. There are multiple reasons to skip this portion of training, and we will discuss a few below.

You did not complete a residency

This is the most straightforward reason to skip a clinically based fellowship. Nearly all clinically based fellowships require successful completion of residency training. If you elected to pursue another career path, such as a traditional research-focused postdoctoral fellowship, then a clinically based fellowship is not an option for you.

Residency training provided sufficient clinical specialization and research time

Some residencies do have built-in dedicated research time that is consolidated and long enough to make significant progress on a research project. For example, if you might choose a surgical residency that has 2-3 years of research time in the middle of the clinical training. It is possible to then apply for a faculty position with protected research time in your specialty after residency without additional fellowship training. Similarly, many pathology residencies are geared toward physician-scientists and have built-in research time that may be adequate to gain independence. Of note, this is not the case with internal medicine or pediatrics. These residencies are too short, and the amount of research time given to residents is not sufficient to establish a research program that would make you competitive for a basic-science–oriented academic faculty position.

You are pursuing a career outside of academia

A minority of MD-PhD graduates complete a residency and then choose to go into a field where they spend either very little or no time on clinical care and academic-based research. These careers might be in the pharmaceutical/device industry, consulting, or government/policy. That is not to say research is not a part of these careers, just that it does not require time in clinical fellowship training to do so.

WHAT IS FAST-TRACKING?

The term fast-tracking or short-tracking most often refers to MD-PhD graduates who take advantage of the American Board of Internal Medicine (ABIM) research pathway. This program allows physician-scientists to complete 24 months of internal medicine residency before starting fellowship, instead of the usual 36 months. However, by utilizing this pathway you must commit to at least 3 years of at least 80% research time during fellowship. This can actually lengthen your training time depending on the subspecialty chosen. Therefore, the term fast-tracking is a misnomer. This program essentially allows an MD-PhD graduate to trade a year of internal medicine residency for a year of research in fellowship. Other specialties (but not all) have similar programs. For example, the Accelerated Research Pathway (ARP) is the equivalent in pediatrics, with 2 years of general comprehensive pediatric training followed by subspecialty fellowship training for a minimum of 4 years. Similarly, pathology has the Physician-Scientist Research Pathway available for serious physician-scientists. This option provides at least one additional year of protected research time, but it does not eliminate any of the core requirements of a pathology residency. If this sounds appealing, you should talk to advisors in the specialty you are considering to find out more about the specifics of each program.

There are pros and cons to utilizing these research pathways. One obvious pro is that if you are very committed to a research-based career, this gives you at least one extra year of protected time to establish your research program and apply for grants or publish more. However, in some cases you are sacrificing a year of clinical training, necessitating that you learn what is required for general comprehensive training in a shorter time period. Therefore, it takes a significant amount of self-awareness and supportive clinical and research mentors to determine if this pathway is right for your career.

A number of residency programs in the United States now have physician-scientist training programs (PSTP) or equivalents. These programs are much more loosely defined than their medical school counterparts, Medical Scientist Training Programs (MSTP). At their core, PSTPs exist to support residents and fellows who are committed to pursuing research-based academic medical careers. This is most similar to the stream of Canadian Royal College accredited Clinician-Investigator Programs (CIP) that allow students flexibility in taking time to perform research during residency without decreasing the length of required clinical training. The structure, size, funding, and design of these programs vary dramatically across institutions, so it is difficult to make generalizations about them. Some of these programs in the United States come with a guarantee of a fellowship spot. For example, if you are planning to apply to hematology/oncology fellowships after completing internal medicine residency, the medical oncology division might guarantee you a spot in their hematology/oncology fellowship if you match at that internal medicine residency program. The program may or may not require you to enter the ABIM research pathway.

HOW TO CHOOSE A FELLOWSHIP PROGRAM

The most important aspect of choosing a fellowship is choosing the specialty. Much like choosing a residency, choosing a subspecialty is a highly personal decision. Factors that go into the decision include your desired work-life balance, how competitive the subspecialty is, and most importantly, whether you enjoy the medical practice of the subspecialty enough to potentially do it for the rest of your career. If you hate reading EKGs, you probably should not go into cardiology!

Once you have settled on a specific field, choosing where to apply is the next decision to make. There is an endless list of factors one might consider, but we will highlight a few that are certainly important. These are geography, clinical training, research training, and post-fellowship placement.

Due to the lengthy nature of the MD-PhD path, most MD-PhD graduates are in their early thirties by the time they apply for fellowship. Many are married and have children or are thinking about having children. Therefore, where a program is located might play a more important part in the decision-making process than it did when choosing an MD-PhD program. Luckily, there are excellent fellowships across North America, so you will likely have several from which to choose.

As stated above, one of the goals of a fellowship is to prepare you for clinical practice in a subspecialty. Therefore, it is important to consider the type of clinical training provided at each program. For example, if you are applying for a nephrology fellowship and are interested in focusing on transplant nephrology, then it would be wise to apply to nephrology programs at large transplant centers, or you might miss the type of clinical exposure and learning you need.

The research time, support, and mentoring provided by a fellowship program can make or break your young career as a physician-scientist. If the program only allows for one to two consecutive months of protected research time, it is going to be challenging to delve into a basic research project and make significant progress. Similarly, if there are no physician-scientists to mentor you, it will be hard to be successful. Some fellowships even provide additional funding to help pay for supplies, travel to conferences, or time in core facilities to support your research activities. This can give you an advantage when it comes to making the most of your protected research time.

Finally, you should look at what type of positions the recent graduates have taken. If you desire a tenure-track position at a research university, but no graduates in the last 10 years from a program to which you are applying have such a position, then it is unlikely you will be able to get a job like that. Fellowship program directors are usually proud of their graduates and happy to share where they landed with you.

CHOOSING A MENTOR

Just as choosing a PhD mentor is potentially more important than choosing a medical school, finding the right fellowship mentor is equally crucial. Therefore, many of the same criteria used to select your PhD mentor (Chapter 10) apply to finding a fellowship mentor, with a few caveats. It is much more likely that your fellowship research will be the focus of your career (particularly early on) than your PhD project. So you should make sure that the research question is something about which you are passionate. Second, after fellowship you will need to differentiate yourself from your mentor, so it is important to have conversations about what aspects of a project you can take with you. Finally, you should use this opportunity to gain a new set of skills. Perhaps your PhD was largely computational, and now you want to gain some more hands-on wet-lab skills. Try to incorporate your desire to learn something new into your mentor search.

TRANSITIONING BACK TO RESEARCH

Just as finishing your PhD and returning to medical school was a challenging transition, so too is transitioning from full-time clinical work to mostly research in fellowship. While you were finishing your medical degree and learning how to be a doctor, scientific progress did not stop. There will likely be multiple new discoveries where you will need to catch up. For example, the use of CRISPR as a gene-editing tool was developed after I completed my PhD, while I was finishing medical school and starting residency. You will need to get used to a new lab, lab mates, and procedures. There will likely be experiments or techniques that you performed with ease as a graduate student on which you now need a refresher, or new equipment with which you must familiarize yourself. Finally, just as it was humbling to go from the "senior" graduate student in a lab to the least knowledgeable person on a medical team, the reverse is also true. When you have completed the majority of your clinical training in fellowship, you are likely prepared for independent clinical practice, but you will probably feel quite behind in research with the transition from the wards back to the lab.

Luckily, the skills you developed to succeed during your PhD, MD, and residency training have prepared you well for the transition. By this time, you will know how to seek help when you are struggling, what learning style works best for you, and how to lean on colleagues, friends, and family to keep you grounded. Unlike the transition to the wards after your PhD, you have done research before, and the abilities and mindset that got you through your PhD will come back and allow you to once again succeed in the research environment. You must be kind to yourself and not be afraid to ask for help or take things slowly at first until you are caught up.

AFTER FELLOWSHIP

After completing a fellowship, most MD-PhD graduates will apply for a job in academic medicine with a research focus. The amount of time devoted to research in these jobs can vary widely. Alternatively, some MD-PhD graduates look for jobs in government, industry, or primarily clinical jobs. Chapter 26 ("Securing Your First job") and Chapter 27 ("Career Choices After Graduation") offer more advice on choosing a career and future on your own terms, as a full-fledged physician-scientist. Often, additional time doing mentored research is necessary before you finally achieve independence as a researcher. This can take many forms. Some MD-PhD graduates will stay at the institution where they completed their fellowship in a non–tenure-track position, often called "instructor." This position will allow them to practice medicine in their specialty independently, while using their non-clinical time to continue their research with their fellowship mentor in order to publish their findings so that they are more competitive for grants or academic jobs at another institution. This "post-fellowship-post-doc" period is ill-defined, and the specifics will vary greatly from institution to institution.

CONCLUSION

Fellowship represents another important transition point in the training and career of MD-PhDs. In many ways, it is MD-PhD "finishing school," where you have to finally land on a specific field of medicine and research that will be the focus of your early career. It will prepare you for independent practice in a subspecialty and set you on the road to independence as a researcher. At the same time, you will be asked to truly live as a physician-scientist, because you will likely have some clinical responsibility even during the research phase. Thus, you'll have to switch back and forth between thinking like a doctor and a scientist multiple times, even in the same day! You will need to make important decisions about where to pursue this extra training and whom to mentor you on this final leg of training. While it requires the same type of hard work and determination that was necessary to complete an MD-PhD training program and residency, it is all highly relevant to your immediate future. These factors combine to make fellowship a critical and enjoyable period in MD-PhD training.

26

Securing Your First Job

Kevin Petrecca • Matthew Dankner

Kevin Petrecca *is a graduate of McGill University's MD-PhD program. He is a neurosurgical oncologist, chief of the Department of Neurosurgery at the McGill University Health Centre, and was appointed as the William Feindel Chair in Neuro-Oncology at McGill University. He also directs an active research laboratory at the Montreal Neurological Institute and Hospital, focused on understanding tumor heterogeneity in brain cancer.*

Matthew Dankner *is a fifth year MD-PhD student at McGill University. He is a Montreal native who graduated from McGill University with a bachelor of science in Honors Anatomy and Cell Biology before joining the MD-PhD program. For his PhD studies, Matthew is involved in basic, translational, and clinical research in the area of metastatic brain tumors, working closely with Dr. Petrecca and his research team.*

INTRODUCTION

The goal of this chapter is to share strategies that will help you secure your first job as a physician-scientist. There are many possible career trajectories for MD-PhDs, and that flexibility is the topic of Chapter 27, but this chapter is meant for those who wish to become physician-scientists in academia.

Preparing for a job can seem far off for students thinking about starting an MD-PhD degree, and even for students who are partway or most of the way to the finish line. The recruitment process is varied. Some students are actively recruited to the institution of their residency early on, whereas others establish networks through collaborators and at conferences to negotiate and land their future position at a different institution. The most important message: Start thinking about this and begin planning as early as possible.

WHAT YOU NEED TO KNOW

- Employment isn't as far off as you think. Start planning early.
- Maintain research productivity during residency.
- Networking now can lead to jobs later.
- Don't feel tied to your home institution.
- Negotiate for circumstances in which you thrive; you'll have other opportunities.

MAINTAINING RESEARCH DURING RESIDENCY

When interviewing for a faculty position, it helps to show research productivity that is impactful, prolific, and up-to-date. You will be expected to propose an independent research program derived from your own self-directed research projects. If you do not continue your research activities between your PhD, as part of an MD-PhD program, and the time when you are searching for an academic position, there will be at least a 5-year gap in research productivity. Given the rapid pace at which research evolves, building on something completed 5 years earlier will likely be less exciting. Continuing research after your PhD, throughout medical school and residency, will allow you to remain at the cutting edge of science and technology. Chapter 24 presented the challenges of integrating research into your residency and proposes methods to overcome them. Bear in mind that continuing research throughout your medical training without compromising your clinical exposure and skills will require a significant amount of effort and time management skills. This will likely be accompanied by a degree of sacrifice, whether it be on your own personal time or other aspects of your life, such as family or hobbies.

POSTDOCTORAL RESEARCH FELLOWSHIP TRAINING

Taking the time for a formal postdoctoral research fellowship immediately before starting your faculty position is highly recommended. This can often be done after your residency in lieu of a clinical fellowship or even in the allotted research time offered within many residency programs. Your considerations in choosing a research fellowship will be similar to those addressed in Chapter 25, which focuses on clinical fellowships, with a few additional concerns. A research postdoc is as much about remaining at the cutting edge of science and publishing high-impact papers as it is about positioning yourself to start your own research program. You may be tempted to skip this step and begin working immediately after residency, but I urge you to strongly consider a postdoc to get your research program up and running and acquire preliminary data that can be used for early grant applications. There is a significant failure rate and the so-called "valley of death" that physician-scientists face if they are not successful in their first grant application cycles. A successful research postdoc will reduce this risk.

When selecting the ideal postdoctoral lab, it is critical that the research project be truly on the cutting edge, allowing you to produce impactful work that can eventually be turned into your own research program that will excite your future colleagues. It's also important to clearly identify, with your future supervisor, the aspects of your project that you will develop in your own research program. It can be difficult to find the perfect scenario, so we urge trainees to begin thinking about this early. This means building strong collaborative connections with researchers around the world, whether through your own research or through conference networking. This process can be initiated as early as during the PhD phase of the MD-PhD program.

WHEN TO START LOOKING AND NETWORKING

Students should start thinking about where they wish to begin their post-training career as early as possible. When interviewing for residency positions, it is not unreasonable to inquire about the anticipated job outlook in your specialty of interest in the coming years. In addition, keeping in touch with collaborators at different institutions will help with this without you even realizing it. Whenever possible, make the effort to get to know people whom you may have an interest in working with as colleagues in the future, and don't keep your career plans a secret.

FINDING THE RIGHT FIT

As an MD-PhD graduate, you will likely be in high demand. Take advantage of this opportunity and allow yourself to be mobile. Even if your home institution wants to recruit you, prioritizing the best environment for your career should be at the top of your list. The institution must support physician-scientists by providing protected time for research, clinical exposure that is directly related to your research area of interest, and a culture of nurturing early-career physician-scientists. You do not have to be the trailblazer facing an uphill battle to exist as a physician-scientist; it is difficult enough of a career path as it is. It is best to find a department with a successful track record of supporting and developing physician-scientists.

One reason for the high failure rate of physician-scientists is that they often agree to sub-optimal offers that do not put them in a strong position for early success. Negotiating a strong startup package and a favorable clinic-research time division is essential for a successful start to your career. When the research programs of early-career physician-scientists do not thrive and they are not able to secure grant funding, they will typically fall back on their clinical practice and ultimately stop research altogether. To minimize this risk, no more than 50% of your time should be allocated to clinical work, with a preference for even less.

The nature of your clinical responsibilities is also important. Your clinical work should be directly in line with your research program. This fulfills the mission of the physician-scientist—to bridge the clinical and research gap for a particular disease or population.

Lastly, starting your research program is as, if not more, challenging than it is for a researcher. You should strive to negotiate for 3–5 years of startup funds for your research program that are equal to or more than that of pure researchers. If you are in the fortunate position of having multiple institutions trying to recruit you, use these issues to leverage for the most favorable offer.

CONCLUSION

Successfully landing a position as a physician-scientist is no easy task. The earlier trainees start to think about what they would like their careers to look like and where they want to work, the better prepared they will be in the recruitment process. Maintaining the flexibility to be mobile will enable you to find the perfect environment to begin your career. The long road to becoming a physician-scientist is full of hard work and challenges. However, this last step also deserves your effort and attention.

27

Career Choices After Graduation

Patrick Williams

Patrick Williams *completed his MD, CM, and PhD at McGill University in 2013. He finished his internal medicine residency at the University of Maryland Medical Center and the Baltimore Veterans Affairs Health Care System, followed by fellowship training in oncology at the MD Anderson Cancer Center in Houston, Texas. He is now a medical director at Genentech, where he leads a number of clinical trials and collaborates with research initiatives in cancer immunotherapy.*

INTRODUCTION

When I first met my PhD supervisor, Jacques Galipeau, who was interviewing me to join his lab, he asked me, "Are you a baker or a cook?" The question was ironic, since I unknowingly had a decade of frozen pizza and cafeteria food in store for me. My supervisor was an MD who had completed two fellowships in the United States to acquire the scientific experience that enabled him to have a successful career practicing medicine while also running a lab.

I didn't appreciate the meaning behind this question until after I returned to the clinic, after completing my PhD and started to take care of patients. The implication behind the question is that medicine is like cooking, while baking is like doing science. When practicing medicine, nothing is a clean, controlled experiment. Your patients are like carrots, onions, and tomatoes: They're never quite the same, and being a good cook isn't simply following a

> **WHAT YOU NEED TO KNOW**
>
> - Build relationships with good mentors, and do not be afraid to reach out. People will open doors for you.
> - Be open-minded about your clinical and research interests. Your dream career might not be what you expected it to be when you started.
> - Do not underestimate the value of your skills and knowledge; it is easy to lose perspective when you're going through your research and clinical training.
> - It is intimidating that your career is what you want to make of it, but you have tremendous job security.
> - Do not hesitate to change course if you are unhappy, as there is always an abundance of options open to you.

recipe, it's knowing what your sauce is supposed to taste like. You have to adjust as you go along. Science requires precision like baking, where small deviations from the protocol can turn your cake into a disappointing pile of failure and sadness.

Manaf Bouchentouf, a postdoc I had the pleasure of working with during my PhD, taught me that the key to learning medicine or doing science had nothing to do with the subject matter I was studying. Training in medicine and research is about creating a mental framework for asking and answering questions, and learning to communicate those answers. Finally, along the same lines, one of my attendings, Philip Mackowiak, made this observation as I was going through my internal medicine residency: "You know, Patrick, what you do is very interesting, because when you're a physician and you see patients, your job is to provide answers, to provide security. When you're a scientist, your job is to ask questions and take that security away." These examples describe what is at the foundation of each individual career, and they made me appreciate the mental gymnastics that come with balancing both roles. This chapter is about finding a career that balances cooking and baking in a way that works for you.

BALANCING TIME BETWEEN MEDICINE AND RESEARCH

The people you will meet throughout your training will look at being an MD-PhD through a different lens, and their perspectives are very telling of where they came from. Manaf's view is that of a PhD: he boiled the experience down to asking questions, writing papers, and presenting data. Philip's view was that of an MD, where a fundamental part of taking care of patients is addressing the patient's disease with the right treatment, and their illness by providing security. Jacques had insights from both (and he liked to cook). But combined medical and scientific training is not always flowers and sunshine. I would hear from some that "MD-PhDs are the future," while others would tell me that going into cancer immunotherapy was "listening to the sirens drawing me out to sea to die" and that "research was a waste of time" for physicians. That being said, cancer immunotherapy was named the journal Science breakthrough of the year in 2013.

The reality is that MD-PhDs have fantastic job security. The worst-case scenario, as cheekily told by Jacquetta Trasler, the MD-PhD program director during my time at McGill, is: "If you fail at research, you quadruple your income. To fail is to gain." What makes going through this career path challenging is that this job security isn't for any one given job. It is very much a game of choose-your-own-adventure. It can be very intimidating to navigate when you don't know what the rules are, when you feel like the rules are stacked against you, or when you don't know what you need to do to win. Your relationships with your mentors are an essential part to figuring this out. I say mentors, plural, because you should have more than one mentor. Each will have a different perspective, and, depending on how much of a cook or a baker you are, you will develop your own opinions on how you want to be an MD-PhD. You will never run into a shortage of good people who will want to help you succeed. Ultimately, having both degrees isn't about being an MD with a PhD, because the whole is greater than the sum of its parts. Each person's career will be highly individualized, balancing values, medicine, and science.

My former fellowship director, Robert Wolff, told me that the trick to succeeding as an MD-PhD comes down to "work-work balance." At face value, this implies that you won't have work-life balance, because taking care of patients and doing research are each full-time jobs.

However, what bears emphasizing here is that the choice that needs to be made is how you want to balance your time between medicine and research. This comes down to how different medical professions and the type of research you do will require your time.

CARVING YOUR CAREER PATH

I didn't appreciate how diverse the career opportunities were for MD-PhDs until I had reached fellowship and had to think about how I was finally going to use my 10-plus years of training. I had aspired to one of the more common scenarios for MD-PhDs, wanting to become an academic physician-scientist, balancing my time between the lab and the clinic. I eventually became a medical director at Genentech, because this was the best opportunity to be at the tip of the immunotherapy spear against cancer. While certain fields have a greater representation of MD-PhDs than others, MD-PhDs can be found in all domains of medicine, and they're not all confined to the lab. As I progressed through my training, it became increasingly clear that everyone forged their path differently. Potential MD-PhDs who are not lab-oriented should not allow the historical association between MD-PhDs and bench research to dissuade them from pursuing careers outside the lab, as several of my friends and former colleagues have taken less conventional routes in psychology, general surgery, ophthalmology, dermatology, and public health. What makes these opportunities more challenging is they can often depend on the insights that you've gained from your experiences. It requires additional legwork to make other people see and care enough about these issues to pay you to do it as your job.

STRATEGIES FOR SUCCESS

To succeed in academia, you need to be "the one person for the one thing" in your institution. There are other roles for MD-PhDs in academia than that of a physician-scientist running a lab and having a clinic. To be a good researcher, you need to have an eye for incongruity, the ability to ask specific questions with testable hypotheses, and the creativity to find solutions. None of this requires you to be in a lab with mice and pipettes. Ultimately, the skill set required to maintain your career will be distinct from the one that got you there. A former mentor, Michael Davies, would half-joke that his early successes were dependent on his technical skills in the lab and that now, later in his career, his lab manager purposefully keeps him away so he doesn't break things.

If you want to succeed with a lab, you'll need an 80/20 lab/clinic split of your time, with no more than one day of clinic per week. This becomes more complicated if you're in a less conventional field like surgery and your technical skills are correlated with the amount of practice you have, but it is not impossible. Certain kinds of research, such as clinical research, may not require the same amount of protected time as bench research; the space between basic science and clinical research is a spectrum from understanding basic biology to conducting translational research to performing clinical trials. Regardless of your role in academia, you will need to "buy your time back," meaning any time you spend outside the clinic needs to compensate for the income the hospital loses because you didn't see patients. This is particularly challenging because funding rates are at record low levels. If you're in Canada, Canadian Institutes of Health Research (CIHR) has undergone several significant changes in the past several years. If you're in Quebec, you may be confronted with certain unwritten rules about the need to acquire training outside the province, as well as PREMs (Plans Regionaux d'Effectifs Medicaux).

At the end of your long training, when the time comes for contract negotiations, you're going to need to carefully compare the offers you receive, because they will be very different. There will be a number of priorities that you will need to balance based on your professional goals and geographic restrictions including, but not limited to: salary, number of days of clinic, number of weeks of inpatient service, operating room (OR) availability, the need for a physician-scientist package to start up your lab or facilitate collaborations, the technological resources available to you within the institution, and the quality of the available mentorship. Some institutions may have a platform ready to go for you to use, whereas others may want you to help build a platform from the ground up. For some positions, your chair may see you only as a warm body to see patients and overburden you with clinical responsibilities that would interfere with your ability to do the research you need to maintain the grants cycle. Others may want to invest in your professional development.

You can expect that top-shelf institutions will be more competitive, by which I mean they'll offer a lower salary, fewer benefits, and demand more in terms of past and future productivity as rewards for the privilege of working there. I strongly recommend that you speak with your mentor(s) about these topics over time to help guide your career, as well as to have a lawyer review your contract before signing anything. As you consider increasingly specialized positions, it will be essential that you consider how each step impacts the next because, for example, the last thing you want is to start a fellowship program that will not offer you the time and opportunities you need to reach the milestones for the job you want, or for your job to set you up for failure by requiring so much time inpatient and outpatient that you can't write grants and do research. The most important resource that you will ever have throughout your training and after is protected time. As you accumulate responsibilities, it will become increasingly important that you balance your priorities, because the reward for good work is more work, not less work. Identify the metrics that you'll be evaluated by early on, and make sure you stay on track to meet those goals. While being a physician-scientist may require you to "get the Nature paper," being a clinical investigator may not.

WORKING IN INDUSTRY

In contrast, the key to success in industry is the ability to adapt. There is tremendous turnover within industry, because people will move between and within companies, and the priorities will change with new leadership. For example, you may specialize in leukemia biology and be a leukemia physician for life while in academia. In industry you may start working broadly in hematology but could transition to solid cancers further down the line based on what your team needs or the opportunities available to you. The transition to industry from academia is abrupt, because the training you've undergone throughout residency and fellowship doesn't really prepare you for what you will do. Everyone I've met or spoken to has told me that it can take over 1 year to get used to the new surroundings. I would liken the experience to being an intern all over again, where you have the theory but need the practical experience of the working with the different roles around you and how you can work with everyone to get your job done.

The companies are much more likely to value your MD than your PhD, but there are positions for scientists within industry. If you want to do research in a lab, the expectations for publications are similar to academia, and there is a regular evaluation for what will continue to be funded. There are companies that will appreciate your ability to read and understand the science, but ultimately what they will inquire about is your experience reading, writing, and conducting clinical trials. Few fellowship programs will grant you this opportunity, which is why many people transition to industry after working for a few years as clinical investigators. Your experience in industry will also vary significantly based on the size of your company. You can generally categorize companies as small, medium, and large, and this will significantly impact your responsibilities and the expectations of the people around you.

My recommendation, if you're interested in a position in industry, is to start at a medium to large pharmaceutical company where you will have adequate mentorship, as you will have the support you need to acquire practical experience interacting with other companies, regulatory bodies in different countries, safety science, operations, and other members in your clinical science team. Once you have joined a company, it is also recommended that you stay there at least 2–3 years, because like academia, it is a small world, and you don't want to develop a reputation as someone that moves around frequently. Taking care of patients is a uniquely rewarding experience, and it bears emphasizing that working in pharma does not necessarily mean you have to abandon your career as a physician. I know several people who have maintained an active clinic and several continue to do, despite having made the jump. They do this while also being able to manage potential conflicts of interest.

CONCLUSION

If you're reading this after getting an MD and are considering enrolling in a PhD program later in your training, it may not be too late for you to do so, but it should also prompt some soul searching. Trying to do bench research like a PhD after completing an MD can be like trying to plug a square peg into a round hole, because the way you're trained to approach and solve problems as an MD is very different from that of a PhD. This isn't to imply that an MD can't learn, that an MD is without value in research, or that a PhD is without value to an MD in or out of academia. The questions you want to ask are: "Why do you want to do this now?" and "Will investing an additional 4 or more years (and the personal life sacrifices and deferred salary that come with that to complete a PhD) alter the course that your career is already on?" There are good answers to these questions, but they are unique to each person, and how you will go about answering them will be different depending on your background.

One of my best friends, David Steffin, has graciously allowed me to share his story with you to illustrate a common struggle. Pediatric oncology is an academic career, and research experience is a common way to be competitive in academia. His time in the lab was often challenging, because he had to rapidly familiarize himself with a very complex field. He had to learn how to conduct experiments, write papers and grants, while also taking care of his patients in the clinic and the hospital. A year later, projects were moving forward, but given his limited research background, he was not sure how he would fit into the field of laboratory science in the long term. He eventually decided against staying in the lab and instead focused on translational research and patient care, which he thoroughly enjoyed. He had gained enough experience to speak the language of both MDs and PhDs. With the biological insights that he acquired, he sufficiently understood CAR T-cell biology to bring his scientific experience to the clinic and translate it to patients. He has since secured a 3 year K12 physician scientist grant and a faculty position as a pediatric hematologist/oncologist conducting CAR T-cell clinical trials in children with relapsed and refractory solid cancers.

While David's is an example of taking the research back to the clinic, Jonathan Cools-Lartigue's is an example of taking medicine to research. He completed his PhD during his surgical residency at McGill, applying his skills to investigate the relationship between the ability for cancer to metastasize and postsurgical infections. The right decision for you will come down to how your medicine informs your science and how your science informs your medicine in a way that lets you stand out and feel fulfilled.

Part VI

Physician-Scientist Wellness

28

Starting a Family During the MD-PhD Program

Guido I. Guberman

Guido I. Guberman *is a fifth-year MD-PhD candidate at McGill University. He is pursuing his PhD in neuroscience at the Integrated Program in Neuroscience. His research focuses on combining novel brain imaging techniques with multivariate statistical analyses to improve diagnostic and prognostic criteria of pediatric concussions.*

INTRODUCTION

The MD-PhD program provides dedicated training time in both medicine and research. Training in one discipline almost inevitably comes at the expense of the other. The long period of training, the daunting demands and expectations, and the high degree of stress are often a deterrent for anyone interested in starting a family. The purpose of this chapter is to dispel that fear and discuss how the MD-PhD path can be compatible with family life. This chapter will outline the challenges and advantages of starting your family during your studies. It will conclude with tips for leading a satisfying career and family life. This chapter is limited by my perspective as a man.

GENERAL CHALLENGES TO STARTING A FAMILY

There are different ways to start a family, which are reflective of different demographic realities. In addition to the approach of naturally conceiving a child with a partner, other ways of starting a family include entering a relationship with a person who has a child, adoption,

WHAT YOU NEED TO KNOW

- Starting a family during the MD-PhD program is possible.
- It requires being aware of the compromises at each stage.
- How supportive a program is for starting a family should be factored in when choosing a school.
- Take time off, take care of your mental health, and develop a work ethic based on efficiency.
- Build a support network, and devote time to your relationship with your partner.

surrogacy, or conception through the use of assisted reproductive technology. Each of these scenarios presents its own challenges, which are far too complex and varied to address in a single chapter. This chapter, which is written from my perspective as a heterosexual cis-gendered male in a relationship with a heterosexual cis-gendered female, presents the challenges associated with having a first child through natural conception. Its scope is therefore limited.

The challenges of starting a family begin in pregnancy. Your partner will start experiencing bodily changes, and research suggests that as a partner, your social and emotional support is beneficial to the mental health of the mother and child. There are different ways of offering support, for instance, by attending all prenatal doctor's appointments, assisting your partner during prenatal classes, and assuming a larger proportion of the household chores. Having a child requires logistical preparation (such as preparing a nursery and making the house childproof). The birth of the baby is also a hectic period. For a vaginal delivery without complications, the length of your partner's hospitalization will be around 48 hours, a period that can be lengthened if any complications arise. The first few months of your baby's life will also likely be intense as you adjust to a new routine. A newborn requires feeding every one to three hours, guaranteeing sleepless nights. This frequency decreases as the child grows. To ensure no health issues arise, frequent visits to the doctor will also be needed. Throughout this process, actively participating in raising your child is critical, especially as your partner recovers from the birthing process. Family life is dynamic, and the challenges of parenthood will evolve as your child grows. For instance, a 5-year-old will require less constant attention than a newborn, but other responsibilities arise at this stage, like finding a kindergarten and a suitable sport for your child.

CHALLENGES TO STARTING A FAMILY DURING THE MD-PhD PROGRAM AND TIPS TO MANAGE THEM

I have repeatedly conversed with individuals interested in the MD-PhD path, and one of the questions that recurs the most is whether it would have been a better idea to wait until the end of my studies to start a family. My first daughter was born seven days before my McGill MD-PhD interview. I knew that sleepless nights and intense periods of study awaited. I was aware that the road in front of me would be challenging, but I also knew I would not have it any other way. My answer is that there is no ideal time to start a family. For some, waiting until after studies may work best, but the truth is that every part of the MD-PhD path, even post-study, can present challenges to starting a family. What is critical is to think ahead and consider what type of challenges you and your family are willing to face, and understand what you are compromising as a consequence. In this part of the chapter, I will outline the potential challenges with each step of study and tips for how to manage them.

Pre-clerkship

Most medical school curricula are divided in two main sections, pre-clerkship and clerkship. The pre-clerkship phase, detailed in Chapter 8 ("Starting Medical School and Integrating Research"), entails regular class time, laboratory sessions, periodic written and practical examinations, and other forms of evaluation. The particular methods of evaluation and the format of class time may vary between universities. Some schools have a pass/fail system of evaluation; others assign grades that go on a permanent transcript. Some schools have regular 8 AM to 5 PM classes, whereas others have case-based learning. The logistics of pre-clerkship medicine are variable and highly relevant for selecting your program when you are interested in starting a family. Some schools strictly require students' presence in the class; others put recordings of the lectures online. Importantly, however, all programs require extensive self-directed work: reviewing for classes, studying for exams, completing exercises, and preparing for laboratory sessions. In addition, even in schools with highly flexible policies regarding class attendance, certain sessions will still be required (written and laboratory exams). The main challenge at this step is to manage this self-directed work and different scheduling obligations with the challenges of family life mentioned above. Take advantage of class recordings if available, obtain notes from classmates in case of family emergencies, and/or let professors know in advance if a doctor's appointment for your child is expected.

During your PhD

The pace of the PhD portion is generally very different. Chapters 11 to 17 gave a more comprehensive overview of this stage. Although coursework is required, it likely occupies a smaller portion of the week. PhD programs require different amounts of courses, but all will have extended periods of time for research activities. As a result, the PhD is usually more flexible with respect to time in comparison to medical school. That is not to say that the workload is smaller; in fact, it may even be larger. However, depending on the nature of your research, your hours are generally more self-determined; it will not necessarily be mandatory to follow a specific schedule. During this period, you can apply for awards, which can provide additional financial security. In some schools, your PhD will be shorter than normal. To compete against individuals with 2–3 additional years of training, higher demands are necessary.

The end of a PhD requires extensive work, and MD-PhD programs have a hard deadline for when to return to medical school. Balancing family life with a suddenly flexible period of training requires a lot of self-directed work, discipline, and organization. More importantly, adaptability is required, given that demands increase exponentially at the end of the degree. In addition, once the PhD stage of the program is completed, a quick change in schedule will take place. Planning ahead for this change is crucial.

Clerkship

Schedules during clerkship (clinical rotations) are drastically different. This phase of learning was the topic of Chapters 18 to 22, but the key points for a prospective parent to know will be reviewed here. Attendance is strictly mandatory and usually inflexible. Rotations tend to be short, between two to four weeks, which makes schedules very variable. Some rotations may have predictable, even short hours, while others may have long hours. Overnight shifts and being on call may be necessary as well. In the latter part of this stage, moving out of town may be required for elective rotations. Taking time off is difficult, and for many schools, your performance reviews during this period are the main method of evaluation when applying to residency. These inflexible, potentially unpredictable, and heavy time demands are the main challenge to starting a family at this stage. Help and collaboration from family is especially important during this period. Your school can offer parental leave of absence, sick leave, and flex days (all discussed later in this chapter). All these options should be considered if starting a family during this stage of your training.

Starting a family after the MD-PhD program

This section is meant to dispel the idea that it is best to wait until after your MD-PhD training to start a family. Chapters 23 to 27 correspond to this part of your career path. Given that

I am not at this stage of my training yet, I will only briefly cover some of the more well-known challenges of starting a family after the MD-PhD program.

All practicing physicians have to pursue some type of postgraduate medical training. The residency period is characterized by strict and often longer working hours. The responsibilities of a resident are much more numerous, and more hours on call are required. A residency may last between 2 and 6 years, and may require moving to another city, province/state, or even country. Support from family and friends will be harder to obtain when you are starting your own family abroad. Furthermore, uprooting your family will also require coordinating with your partner and ensuring the move is not detrimental to their career, if applicable.

Some individuals who pursue a career as a physician-scientist may wish to complete a postdoctoral (postdoc) or a clinical fellowship. Postdocs tend to be short, although they can be prolonged, depending on the nature of the research and funding availability. In addition, whether it is a clinical or a research postdoctoral fellowship, it is generally suggested that it take place at a hospital/laboratory in a different institution from the one where the majority of the training took place. This expectation is usually greater for postdoctoral/clinical fellowships than for residency, so again, the challenges of starting a family far from your support network are important to consider. Furthermore, applying for positions as a physician-scientist will be important at this stage and might require yet another move.

Lastly, if you started the MD-PhD program after an undergraduate degree, and you plan to complete a 4-year PhD, a 5-year residency, and a 2-year postdoc without any breaks anywhere in between, you will be approximately 37 when you finish your studies. The physical stress of having a child and starting a family has been mentioned earlier, but it is important to note that the stress only becomes more difficult as stamina decreases with age. The risk of adverse birth outcomes also increases with paternal age. The challenges for women can of course be much different. In addition, if you have managed to obtain a position as a physician-scientist, you will be working diligently to establish your laboratory and clinical practice. Doing so will entail conducting multiple studies, publishing frequently, traveling for conferences, setting up collaborations, competing for grants, training students, building your patient base, and perfecting your skills. This period is likely to be intense and stressful.

LEAVES OF ABSENCE

Each school has its own policies regarding leaves of absence. For anyone interested in starting a family during the program, it will be important to become well-acquainted with the policies regarding absences and leaves. For example, at McGill, there are three types of absences during the MD portion: short-term (half a day to five consecutive calendar days), medium-term (six consecutive calendar days to eight weeks), and long-term (more than eight weeks). For each type of absence, there are different reasons for requesting leave.

During the PhD portion of the program, requests for parental leave are submitted in writing to the department, which forwards the request to Enrollment Services. This leave can be granted for a period of up to 52 weeks, or approximately 12 months. If a student taking this leave has external funding, the student needs to contact the agency granting the funding to learn about their policies. For instance, in Canada, according to the Tri-Agency Research Training Award Holder's Guide, trainees can obtain a paid leave of

12 months maximum. Becoming well-acquainted with the policies governing leaves of absence at each school is an important part of planning to start a family.

FLEXIBILITY AND ORGANIZATION: A DELICATE BALANCE

With the presented configuration, one can foresee a period of flexibility when transitioning from preclinical medicine to graduate school, which can certainly be advantageous when adjusting to family life. On the other hand, being away from medicine for 4 years may make transitioning back to medical school after the PhD harder. In other schools, the PhD portion takes place at the beginning of the program. Transitioning to clinical medicine might be easier, but it makes the preclinical medicine part less ideal for starting a family, since it will be immediately followed by a far more intense period. Once again, all of these factors are important to consider. All of them can be overcome, but all come at a cost. More time-demanding periods will likely keep you away from family, but they may also be more predictable and thus easier to organize. More time-flexible periods can allow you to spend more time with family, but organizational skills will certainly be required. One should consider these demands and assess one's own qualities, needs, and priorities when deciding when and where to start a family.

TIPS TO LEADING A SATISFYING CAREER AND FAMILY LIFE

As a result of raising a daughter while starting my MD-PhD studies, I have come up with a list of tips that might help when trying to start a family during the MD-PhD training. The objective of these suggestions is not only to integrate family life with work and study, but to enjoy each part as much as possible.

Take time off

I knew early on in my studies that integrating family and work meant first determining what kind of career and family life I wanted. It is easy to determine what a successful work life signifies for an MD-PhD: frequent publishing, excelling in clinical duties, and obtaining grants. But a successful family life is more ambiguous. For me, it meant being able to regularly spend time with my daughter. It meant ensuring that she never saw me as absent, only as busy. Practically, it meant taking off most weekends to do something special with her, take her to the park or to the pool, or go hiking. And that is my first suggestion: take time off. Reserve a regular amount of your time to spend with your family. Turn off your computer and take the time to be present with your family. One may think that research productivity will be increased by simply working more hours, but fewer hours spent working well are worth more than many spent working poorly. As difficult as it might be to accept, even with our busy schedules, not all of our time is indispensable for work.

Build a support network

Shortly after my first daughter was born, I started medical school. Being a father and a medical student both required their own adjustment periods. I needed to adapt to intense work schedules, baby food, frequent examinations, sleepless nights, anatomy labs, and diapers. Without the help I received from family and especially from my spouse, adjusting to these changes simultaneously would have been impossible. That is my second suggestion: Build a support network (i.e., surround yourself with people who can help you). It might require asking family members to babysit or cook, or asking classmates to send you their notes if you have to miss class. Seeking advice from other students with children can also help. Nobody is expected to raise a child or to become a physician-scientist completely alone, and the same applies for people doing both.

Invest in your relationship with your partner

There are only so many hours in a day. If you are raising a child with a partner, it is often easy to invest all your time in that child, often at the cost of spending time with your partner. For physician-scientists, given our time limitations, it is even easier to neglect our relationships with our partners. When one thinks of balancing family with work, one often thinks of ensuring that you spend enough time with your children. It may sound obvious, but to lead a rewarding family life, your relationship to all members of your family must be healthy, especially with your partner. I know for me, family life feels at its best when my relationship with my partner feels at its best. So, my third suggestion is to ensure you invest time and effort in your relationship with your partner, if this is applicable to you. That may require occasionally leaving your children with family to do activities as a couple.

Modify your work ethic to prioritize efficiency

When I started medical school, I had just finished my bachelor's degree. I was keen, energetic, and eager to learn everything. Despite having taken full workloads in the past while balancing extracurricular activities, I was not fully prepared for the pace of preclinical medicine. The amount of information being thrown at you is excessive, and it is easy to feel that you cannot grasp all of it. Learning in this excess of information should teach you how to be selective with the information you retain. Several schools have pass-fail systems because they recognize that different people have different life circumstances. You will have many opportunities to review the material as you start encountering patients. My fourth suggestion is to modify your work ethic to prioritize efficiency. For instance, if your school has a pass-fail system, do not aim for a 95% in an exam where the grade does not matter and will not determine whether or not you will be a good doctor. Take that time to get started on research or to spend time with family. It is important to do your best and prioritize learning, but remember that you are starting the rest of your life at the same time.

Take care of your mental health

One may think that being accepted into an MD-PhD program is the hardest step of the training path, and that once this milestone is achieved, the feeling of fulfillment will automatically signify happiness. The truth is quite the opposite. The physician-scientist path is paved with the intense time demands of medical school, the constant pressure of research productivity, and the overbearing feelings of inadequacy that stem from being surrounded by highly achieving and intelligent people and having to compete against individuals who work full time in either of your two fields. These challenges are intense and prolonged, the entire experience can be isolating, and your motivation can understandably wane over time. It is entirely normal for this career path to take a toll on your mental health, and starting a family, which comes with its own set of important demands and expectations, may add onto this stress. My final piece of advice is therefore to take care of your mental health. Identify what keeps you well, and make sure to invest time in yourself. Reach out for help if you feel it is necessary, from family, friends, and/or mental health professionals. An entire chapter, perhaps an entire book would be necessary to adequately cover this topic. But suffice it to say, leading a rewarding physician-scientist and family life is as much about taking care of your patients, your research, and your family as it is about taking care of yourself.

CONCLUSION

I hope the advice presented in this chapter helps anyone interested in starting a family while training to become a physician-scientist. The medical and research field will need you, and starting a family should not be the factor that deters you from pursuing an MD-PhD degree. The training path is long and arduous, but you should not sacrifice starting a family for it either. It is challenging but certainly possible to do both.

29

Gender and Physician-Scientist Training

Maya Overby Koretzky • Caitlin Bowen

Maya Overby Koretzky *is a fifth-year MD-PhD student at Johns Hopkins University. Her PhD research is in history of medicine, and focuses on the long history of social determinants of health and the politics of public hospital medicine in the late nineteenth- and early twentieth-century American South. Her previous work has focused on this history of HIV/AIDS and the ethics of brain death and organ transplantation. Maya earned her BA in history from Cornell University in 2013 and worked as a fellow in the Department of Bioethics at the National Institutes of Health prior to starting medical school.*

Caitlin Bowen *is a fifth-year MD-PhD student at Johns Hopkins University. Her PhD research is in human genetics and focuses on the use of genetic and environmental modifiers to understand the molecular mechanisms of rare cardiovascular diseases. Prior to medical school, Caitlin earned her BS in biological engineering from Cornell University and worked as a fellow in the National Heart, Lung, and Blood Institute at the National Institutes of Health.*

INTRODUCTION

Many women and gender-minority students considering, admitted to, or matriculated in combined-degree programs have at one point or another expressed apprehension that their gender will negatively affect their training.

> ### WHAT YOU NEED TO KNOW
>
> - Gender disparity remains at all levels of physician-scientist training.
> - Many institutions are committed to increasing gender parity in the physician-scientist workforce.
> - Despite the national gender gap in physician-scientist training, many women and gender-minority students apply to and thrive in MD-PhD training programs and their physician-scientist careers.
> - There are few gender-specific considerations in dual-degree training. Aspects of the dual degree that have often been characterized as women's issues, such as length of training, are considerations that affect people of all genders.
> - Dual-degree candidates may benefit from identifying and working with peer and faculty mentors who share their gender or other identities and should take advantage of the support available at each level of their training.

While it is true that a gender disparity remains for applications to and enrollment in MD-PhD training, despite near gender parity in MD and biomedical PhD programs, efforts are underway at many institutions to change this pattern by committing to train and support a gender-diverse field of scientists, physicians, and physician-scientists. Many women apply to, matriculate in, and complete combined-degree programs and go on to have fruitful research and clinical careers. As a growing number of individuals identify along the gender spectrum, it is likely that the number of gender-minority dual-degree candidates will also increase in future years. Program directors increasingly understand gender diversity more broadly, and issues that have been previously identified as women's concerns in MD-PhD training, such as length of training and the desire to have a family, are recognized more often as important for people of all gender identities.

While modern physician-scientist training is more accessible than ever to women and gender-minority students, there unfortunately remain persistent influences and biases toward the non-male physician-scientist in academia and the world at large. This chapter will address some of these concerns, highlight current research, and provide practical advice for women and gender minorities at all stages of the MD-PhD training pathway, from application and admissions to residency and fellowship training.

APPLYING FOR MD-PhD TRAINING

Relatively few prospective medical students apply to combined MD-PhD programs in the United States, despite a high number of matriculating medical students reporting an interest in being significantly involved with research during their career. Furthermore, gender disparity remains in enrollment in MD-PhD programs, despite the gender parity observed separately in both MD and PhD training programs for many years.

Editorial pieces and studies have provided a number of possible hypotheses for why fewer women apply to MD-PhD training programs [1,2,3,4,5]. The reasons offered include: challenges of combining MD-PhD training and furthering a physician-scientist career with family and childbearing, that women feel they have to be better than their male counterparts to be seen as equals, that women are not being encouraged to become physician-scientists, and a lack of role models for women aspiring to be physician-scientists and academic researchers. However, many of these concerns also arise for women who aspire to be physicians and biomedical scientists through either the MD or PhD pathways, yet they apply to and matriculate at these programs at rates comparable to men.

Recent work has begun to understand and address the gender disparity in MD-PhD applications [3].

- Analysis of application trends stratified by medical school ranking and gender revealed that the difference between the percentage of male and female Medical Scientist Training Program (MSTP) applications to a given program was significantly greater as the school rank became more competitive, a trend not observed among MD applications to the same programs.
- Research suggests that the discrepancy in female applicants to MD-PhD programs isn't due to a general trend in applications being stronger for males at top-ranked programs. Women may have, in general, stronger applications than men at highly ranked schools.

- There is no correlation between the percentage of female applicants and the percentage of female students, suggesting that women enroll at similar rates across many programs despite differences in the proportion of applications from female candidates based on program rank and prestige.

This research suggests that some of the challenges facing women who aspire to be physician-scientists occur early in their career trajectory and that the challenges and roadblocks to gender equality are not necessarily inherent to the MD-PhD pathway (such as program length and combining a future career with family and childbearing). Rather, they lie in the idea that women may feel they have to be better than their male counterparts to be seen as equals[3]. Although program length and combining a future career with family are often cited as roadblocks to MD-PhD program applications, they are not inherently gender-specific challenges.

Advice for the application process

While research and interventions into improving the application climate for female and gender-minority students remain ongoing, we would like to provide some advice for women or gender minorities in the application process.

If you find yourself discouraged by faculty or other mentors on the basis of your gender, identify other mentors who will be more supportive of your goals. Many physician-scientists are more than willing to provide advice or serve as informal mentors even before you are accepted to an MD-PhD program. If you are interested in a dual-degree program, a great way to build a mentorship network and learn more about MD-PhD options is by identifying individuals with your background, research interests, and/or gender identity at your institution or in your geographic area and emailing them to introduce yourself. That said, it is important to obtain mentoring from a diversity of supportive sources.

If you have questions about your application or your strength as an applicant, reach out to MD-PhD program directors or current MD-PhD students. Contact information for many of these individuals can be found online easily. Applicants tend to gather information about MD-PhD programs from sources that tend to be informal and social in nature, such as research mentors, peers, and the Internet, which may not have accurate information or be free from implicit biases[6]. You cannot make an informed decision without the right information.

Once you reach the interview stage of the process, remember that you are interviewing the programs you visit just as much as they are interviewing you. It may be a good idea to research what opportunities and support each program has for female or gender-minority students prior to your interview. While interviewing, it is appropriate to ask current students with your gender identity about their experiences, and to consider if the program has faculty who could provide mentorship to you in this area.

Be aware that programs are legally not allowed to ask personal questions, such as questions about your relationship status, sexual orientation, physical appearance, plans to get pregnant, or gender identity. If you are asked these kinds of questions on your interview, in most circumstances it is a good idea to mention it to current students or to the program director (if you feel comfortable). Programs do not want their interviewers to ask these kinds of questions, and it should not negatively impact you if you choose not to answer them.

MEDICAL SCHOOL CONSIDERATIONS

Since 2002, men and women have enrolled in medical school in near-equal numbers. In 2017, more than half of all matriculants to medical school were female, and starting in 2018, more than half of all applicants to medical school were female.

During the clinical years of medical school, you will work with a wide variety of faculty, support staff, and patients. Older faculty acting as clinical supervisors on the wards are frequently male. While some specialties may have less gender parity than others, you should not feel pressured to avoid or go into any particular specialty based on your gender identity. If you are female or female-presenting, it is still not uncommon to be mistaken for nursing staff by patients or other members of the care team while on the wards. Clearly displaying your medical student badge and wearing your white coat consistently help to avoid any such misidentification.

Should you encounter harassment or gender discrimination on the wards (or in the classroom), most medical schools have a designated office where you can report your experience. It is a good idea to identify this office early in your training so that you can easily find it if a situation arises later on that you need to report.

Professional medical, subspecialty, and scientific organizations will often have large annual meetings that have breakout sessions for trainees on gender, discrimination, and professional development. Be on the lookout for these sessions and mentoring resources, and become involved as a trainee on a national level if you are passionate about improving gender representation in your professional medical field.

GRADUATE SCHOOL CONSIDERATIONS

More than ever before, women are enrolling in PhD programs for biomedical sciences and nontraditional science fields. However, since this gender parity is relatively recent and there is a significant drop off in percentage of women within each level in academic medicine (often referred to as "the leaky pipeline"), the faculty and administration of your graduate program may not be as representative or diverse.

It is important to talk to students in each graduate program that you are considering about their personal experiences and get an idea of the administrative support for women and gender-minority students. Ask program directors about the university resources available for supporting students, particularly with regards to reporting and curtailing gender-based discrimination or misconduct on the part of faculty or other graduate students.

Your experience in graduate school will also depend highly on the mentor you choose and the research environment in which you work on a day-to-day basis. Relying on the experiences and advice of others will be critical when choosing a mentor.

Be sure to talk with older students about their experiences in the lab and with the mentor, particularly in times of difficulty or stress. Also check with your MD-PhD and PhD program directors when you are considering different labs, as they will often have valuable institutional memory regarding previous students' successes and challenges.

While your graduate advisor may be a go-to for sound scientific advice, more likely than not their experiences may not exactly reflect your individual experiences and training.

It is important to identify other people that can mentor you in other capacities, whether it is physician-scientist career mentoring, work-life balance mentoring, or anything else that might come up. These people can be postdoctoral or clinical fellows, lab managers, members of your thesis committee, or people outside your field. Most successful physician-scientists can name multiple clinical and scientific mentors who supported them in their training. It is also important to identify sources of support outside the research environment, whether they are student peers, family, friends, or partners.

RESIDENCY AND FELLOWSHIP CONSIDERATIONS

When it comes time to apply to residency and fellowships, often the advice of your medical school peers will remain true for you as an MD-PhD applicant as well. It is important to remember that the residency training period is for clinical training, so your clinical years will have a larger impact on your success than your research years from your MD-PhD training.

As an MD-PhD applicant, you may be a few years older than your MD-only peers. As such, it may be important to inquire about program support for childcare (if you already have children), or parental leave policies (if you or your partner are planning on having children). Some programs may also have support for your partner, who will have to relocate to wherever you match, including housing referrals or employment assistance. These considerations regarding childcare support are relevant for individuals of all gender identities who are planning on or already have families.

LENGTH OF TRAINING

While length of training has often been emphasized as a consideration for women in MD-PhD programs, this consideration impacts dual-degree candidates of all gender identities. Length of training is important for anyone who would like to start a family during the years of their MD-PhD training, but it is also a consideration for people who are caring for older family members or have other important commitments outside of their careers.

Life continues to happen while you are working toward your dual degree. Many students choose to think of the MD-PhD training as the first stage of their career, rather than simply a training phase. Framing the MD-PhD in this way is a useful illustration of the fact that each student needs to consider their own individual work-life balance, not only once they have an established career, but also while they are working toward their dual degree. For this reason, the location of the training program is an important consideration for many people who are choosing between programs, as is asking program directors about what they do to support students of all gender identities who elect to have families while in training.

CONCLUSION

A gender disparity remains at all levels of physician-scientist training. However, many institutions are committed to increasing gender parity in the physician-scientist workforce, and gender should not be considered a barrier for those interested in applying to or matriculating in MD-PhD programs. Dual-degree candidates may benefit from identifying and working with peer and faculty mentors and should take advantage of the support available for women and gender-minority students at each level of their training. Aspects of the dual degree that have historically been characterized as women's issues, such as length of training, are considerations that affect people of all genders, and despite the national gender gap in physician-scientist training, many women and gender-minority students apply to and thrive in MD-PhD training programs and their physician-scientist careers.

Further Resources

American Medical Women's Association
American Physician Scientist Association
Association of Women in Science and Medicine
Graduate Women in Science
Medical Student Pride Alliance
American Association of University Women

References

A portion of this chapter was reproduced from Bowen CJ, Kersbergen CJ, Tang O, Cox A, Beach MC. Medical school research ranking is associated with gender inequality in MSTP application rates. BMC Med Educ. 2018;18(1):187. doi:10.1186/s12909-018-1306-z under the terms of the Creative Commons Attribution 4.0 International License http://creativecommons.org/licenses/by/4.0/. The only changes made were editorial.

1. Andrews NA. The other physician-scientist problem: where have all the young girls gone? Nat Med. 2002;8(5):439–41.

2. Harding CV, Akabas MH, Andersen OS. History and outcomes of 50 years of physician scientist training in medical scientist training programs. Acad Med. 2017;92(10):1390–1398.

3. Bowen CJ, Kersbergen CJ, Tang O, Cox A, Beach MC. Medical school research ranking is associated with gender inequality in MSTP application rates. BMC Med Educ. 2018;18(1):187.

4. Milewicz DM, Lorenz RG, Dermody TS, Brass LF. Rescuing the physician-scientist workforce: the time for action is now. J Clin Invest. 2015;125(10):3742–7.

5. Cox CL. Balancing Research, Teaching, Clinical Care, and Family: Can Physician-Scientists Have it All? J Infect Dis, 2018;218(1):32–35.

6. Kersbergen CJ, Bowen CJ, Dykema AG, Koretzky MO, Tang O, Beach MC. Student Perceptions of M.D.-Ph.D. Programs: A Qualitative Identification of Barriers Facing Prospective M.D.-Ph.D. Applicants, Teach Learn Med, 2020;1:1–10.

30

Present and Future Roles of Physician-Scientists in Society

Seema Kacker • Justin Lowenthal

Seema Kacker *is a seventh-year MD-PhD candidate at Johns Hopkins University. Seema recently completed her PhD in health economics, with a focus on consumer behavior in the context of zero pricing. She is a senior fellow on the corporate partnerships/business development team at Johns Hopkins Technology Ventures and an ambassador for Breakout Labs, a philanthropic fund focused on investing in early-stage, deep-science companies. She is currently completing her third year of medical school. Prior to the MD-PhD program, Seema completed a bachelor of science in economics from the Massachusetts Institute of Technology and worked for the Abdul Latif Jameel Poverty Action Lab in rural India.*

Justin Lowenthal *is a seventh-year MD-PhD candidate at Johns Hopkins University. His PhD research is in biomedical engineering and centers on using stem cells, genetics, developmental biology, and tissue engineering techniques to model cardiac development and genetic heart disease. Prior to medical school, Justin completed a bachelor of science in biomedical engineering from Yale University and a certificate in bioethics at*

WHAT YOU NEED TO KNOW

- Increasingly, MD-PhD graduates are pursuing postgraduate clinical training and careers with an increased focus on clinical medicine.
- While much of the research conducted by physician-scientists continues to be basic and translational biomedical research, a growing number pursue research in public health, social sciences, and humanities.
- "Habitats" of physician-scientists are becoming more varied; while many report expecting to pursue full-time academic positions, transitions to industry, government, consulting, and other nonacademic paths later in careers are becoming more common.
- Clinical specialties being pursued by physician-scientists, and with it the associated research questions impacting clinical care, are becoming more diverse, with increasing numbers choosing to train outside of typical internal medicine, pediatrics, pathology, or neurology paths and within more procedural specialties.
- The MD-PhD pool is becoming more demographically diverse. This diversity in background and appearance brings with it a diversity in the types of research questions being asked. Furthermore, the breadth of these research questions has expanded the scope of possible physician-scientist careers.

the National Institutes of Health. He has been heavily involved in medical student leadership as well as health policy and social justice advocacy work, frequently contributing to op-eds and policy discussions around emerging biotechnologies and the pricing of prescription drugs in Washington, D.C.

INTRODUCTION

Historically, physician-scientist programs have aimed to produce academic physicians who effectively combine basic science research with clinical practice. The motivation behind this particular combination was that each component would naturally benefit the other. Research conducted by these physicians would be informed by their clinical experience and ability to identify gaps in our capacity to care for patients, and would in turn allow them to provide better patient care and advance our capacity to treat disease and care for patients with new insights and better technology.

In recent years, however, the proportion of graduates from these programs who pursue career paths falling outside of this traditional framework has increased. As a result, the social roles being played by physician-scientists have evolved. A vast array of diverse physician-scientist careers now exists. The unique integrated training of physician-scientists makes them poised to help tackle the multifaceted and complex challenges of improving human health. The very nature of MD-PhD training requires wearing multiple hats, balancing competing priorities, serving multiple constituencies, and acting at the nexus of multidisciplinary projects. Through these experiences, physician-scientists develop an armamentarium of skills that can be used to shape and guide the broader health system and public policy landscape. The professional opportunities available to MD-PhDs span the entire health care system, with physician-scientists playing critical roles in health policy and administration, industry research and development, and biotech startups, for example.

In this chapter, we review recent trends in the professional paths taken by graduates of MD-PhD programs, discuss the multiple factors that may be contributing to these changes, and reflect on how the broader social role of physician-scientists may continue to develop.

CHANGING MIXTURES OF CLINICAL SERVICE AND RESEARCH PURSUITS

Research has traditionally been the focus of physician-scientist training programs and a referenced measure of program success. In fact, an 80/20 division of research to clinical effort is often cited as an optimal mix. However, the collaborative nature of medical research allows clinicians with research expertise to complete projects within larger research endeavors. This provides an opportunity to do research with a primary focus on clinical care. While most MD-PhD graduates are spending some time doing research, this varies across the workplace environment. The average research effort of physician-scientists is significantly higher among those working in industry or research institutes, as compared to full-time academia, and significantly higher among full-time academics as compared to those in private practice. Research effort also varies by specialty. It is generally lower in family medicine and surgery compared to neurology, internal medicine, pediatrics, and pediatric neurology.

Much of the research being conducted by physician-scientists is basic science and translational work, although many investigators are pursuing clinical science more directly, including patient-oriented research and health services research. A growing number of MD-PhDs with graduate training in social sciences and humanities is also leading to increased research conducted through these approaches. Even if trained in a basic science field, investigators may choose to apply their scientific approaches to other types of research questions. This may be partly a result of the limited amount and changing sources of research funding, particularly if those funding sources more often require direct clinical applications. Patient-oriented areas of research may also be easier to combine with clinical commitments, as they often require less infrastructure or other resources to set up, may be more flexible, and can be easier to align with clinically relevant problems. Clinical research based on patient records, for example, may be easier to conduct remotely and with limited funding, as compared to a basic science project requiring a lab, equipment, and trained staff.

Seamlessly combining research and clinical practice is increasingly challenging for physician-scientists and may not always be supported in our current economic climate. Public research funding is limited, but in addition, hospital systems are increasingly financially constrained. This would suggest that hospitals may encourage physicians to generate short-term revenue from clinical operations, rather than investing in longer-term benefits through potentially costly research. Without institutional support for research, it may be difficult for physician-scientists to effectively and efficiently leverage their research training.

CHANGING HABITATS OF PHYSICIAN-SCIENTISTS

Physician investigators are typically associated with academic institutions. Traditionally, the majority of physician-scientists have worked in academia, while far fewer medical school graduates pursue this path, particularly among women. These estimates do vary by choice of specialty, but have declined slightly over time, along with an increase in the proportion of trainees choosing to work in private practice or other workplace environments.

Interestingly, physician-scientists often decide to pursue alternative careers later in training or after starting a job in academia. Some individuals who begin careers as full-time academics transition over time to being part-time academics, working in private practice, working in industry, or working at federal or non-federal research institution.

This is particularly true among trainees who choose to forego postgraduate clinical training. While these graduates would have traditionally pursued academic careers as full-time investigators, it is becoming increasingly difficult to consistently obtain the funding support required and to find appointments in academic departments that do not expect them to provide clinical service.

Multiple factors could lead to a decrease in trainees pursuing full-time academic careers. Notably, the time to MD-PhD degrees has lengthened, as has the time between graduation and the first permanent position. Lengthier training processes mean that trainees are older when they begin stable, established careers, and thus that income would be further delayed for these graduates. This could affect career choice, particularly if alternative nonacademic paths may be more financially attractive than academic positions. Furthermore, for some trainees, the importance of lifestyle and other considerations in these decisions may increase over time, potentially decreasing the likelihood of choosing to pursue a career as an academic.

Simultaneously, alternative paths are becoming increasingly appealing to physician-scientists, particularly if they allow for similar types of problem-solving and innovation without the constraints of academia. In addition, there are a growing number of biotech startup incubators and innovation-friendly cities, leading to increased and more diverse opportunities for physician-scientists coming out of training. Careers in industry, consulting, law, or finance may also be possible.

Veering slightly away from traditional academic paths will likely not change the research contributions of physician-scientists, as most trainees continue to be involved in some form of research even outside of academia. The scope of where this type of work is done, however, has broadened. This could lead to increased efficiency in the translation of research and an increased range of possible approaches and problems being addressed.

CHANGING DISTRIBUTION OF CLINICAL SPECIALTIES FOR PHYSICIAN-SCIENTISTS

Another noticeable trend among physician-scientists who do choose to practice medicine is a change in the distribution in choices of clinical specialty. Traditionally, there have been just a few clinical specialties that were thought to be most compatible with conducting research. The range of specialties being chosen is expanding, however, growing beyond internal medicine, neurology, pathology, and pediatrics. In recent years, there has been an increase in the proportion of MD-PhDs choosing to train in dermatology, emergency medicine, radiology, and radiation oncology, with some evidence of increases in OB/GYN and surgical subspecialties as well.

This trend is likely attributable to multiple factors. These other specialties may have become more accommodating to research-inclined physicians, offering dedicated research time, even at the residency and fellowship levels. In some ways, these specialties may also have more unexplored research questions, which may make them more compelling to curious investigators and more attractive to high-quality researchers. However, research effort among physician-scientists in some of these specialties is often lower than in medicine or other more traditional specialties.

A changing distribution of specialties may also be associated with changes in the demographic distribution of graduating physician-scientists. For example, older graduates who may be concerned with obtaining an established career as soon as possible may pursue specialties with shorter residency programs, those for which the time to obtain a permanent position is shorter, or those that seem most financially appealing.

The evolution of clinical specialties on which physician-scientists are focused suggests that an appreciation for the applicability of this type of multifaceted training is broadening. This will hopefully mean that clinical areas and specific diseases that may have been relatively neglected will experience more growth and innovation. More broadly, the increasing scope of specialty choice suggests that the overall image of what it means to be a physician scientist is changing.

PHYSICIAN-SCIENTISTS DIVERSIFYING

Physician scientist programs are increasingly diverse, both in demographic background and in chosen research areas of focus. Still, barriers to entering these career paths are significant, particularly among typically underrepresented racial/ethnic minorities and women. These barriers often begin at the point of initial application to MD-PhD programs for a variety of reasons, including misconceptions often communicated by undergraduate advisors about MD-PhD training. Caucasian men still dominate the composition of most MD-PhD programs and physician-scientist tracks, both in the applicant pool and those ultimately selected.

However, the overall pool of physician-scientists, both in practice and in training, is indeed diversifying. With increasing diversity in the MD-PhD training population comes increased diversity in the overall physician-scientist pool, increasing representation of women and underrepresented minority groups. With that diversity comes an increased sensitivity to the perspectives and needs of these populations. Moreover, the increased diversity of demographics and inclusion of a larger variety of socioeconomic backgrounds are among several factors leading to increased diversity in research areas—the particular biological questions, disease mechanisms, and communities/populations of focus in that research—that trainees pursue. Among those physician-scientists who choose to pursue some element of research, the specific research areas of focus have broadened to include diseases of particular relevance to underprivileged and vulnerable populations, for example, and research questions targeted toward reducing health disparities. Physicians are more able to promote evidence-based clinical decision making, health policy, and public health intervention in particular areas and for particular groups of patients for which it has been historically lacking (e.g., health of pregnant women; health of uninsured, undomiciled, or undocumented populations).

In addition to diversification of research areas and questions within biological sciences (more traditional wet lab as well as computational research areas), an increased proportion of physician-scientists now study fields outside of basic science, including public health, health services research, bioethics/medical ethics/philosophy of science, history of medicine, medical anthropology, and other social sciences or humanities. This can be partially attributed to a broader understanding that social sciences, population epidemiology, and health economics add value. They are ultimately research areas that can impact health and patient care in ways just as, if not more, significant than the study of basic biological and disease mechanisms.

These trends have contributed to an overall shift in the image of a "physician-scientist" and the perception of their typical roles in medicine and society. Physician-scientists are increasingly involved in activities outside of research labs and clinic hallways, taking on new roles in health policy, health services research, education, communication, and administration. This is likely to benefit scientific research, because solving complex problems is often done most effectively with diverse teams.

GROWTH OF NON-TRADITIONAL ROLES IN SOCIETY

Accompanying and in part informed by the aforementioned four trends is a broader re-imagining of the physician-scientist, with changing perceptions of roles that MD-PhDs can fill, or in some case should be more encouraged to pursue, to contribute to the positive good. Outside of roles providing clinical care at the individual level or pursuing biomedical research at a more macro-level, the changing makeup of MD-PhD programs and shifts in areas of clinical and research interests pursued during training naturally lead toward physician-scientists filling roles that are more varied, including shaping of the broader health system:

- More diverse areas of research and focus in academia and industry
- Diversified clinical foci
- Leaders and administrators for medical institutions and universities
- Leaders of government institutions/departments related to health, medicine, science, tech, public health, social justice, and human rights

- Leaders in the practice and theory of medical education, including efforts to include new scientific and social/advocacy topics in medical school curricula
- Pursuing business and entrepreneurship related to biotechnology, including startup companies, corporate leadership, and venture capital/investing/finances
- Thought leaders in public policy, philosophy of science, and bioethics, including the ethics of emerging medical technologies and new clinical dilemmas
- Roles in communication (journalism, digital media, writing, and social media) that improve public understanding of science and medicine (including ethics and social implications therein)
- Roles in policy and politics, including as politicians, civic leaders, and legislators; government and campaign consultants on health and science issues; broader efforts at civic engagement, advocacy, and activism in the nonprofit and social justice spheres
- Expertise in law and intellectual property conveyed through consulting and expert-witness testimony
- Leading efforts to safeguard human rights globally

Some of the above areas are indeed seeing increased infusions of physician-scientists, whereas others have been noted as areas where more physician-scientist participation would be desirable. Overall, with growing recognition of the importance of public policy, climate and environment, social forces, and economic factors affecting patient care and public health more generally, there is a broadened sphere of issues that are thought to be within the realm of physicians.

In some cases, these may be a broadening of the responsibility of physicians in society (an external stimulus), but in others it is a broadening of areas that physician-scientists are motivated and equipped to address (an internal stimulus). Areas of research and public policy, including population health, climate change, nutrition, and violence/trauma were not previously thought of as in the physician's domain; the individual relationship between a doctor and a patient has long been held sacrosanct and prioritized above population-level (let alone political) considerations.

However, with societal change has come a recognition that physician-scientists can play many diverse and important roles. They are scientists poised to adapt to change as experts in evidence, empirical data, and analytical thinking. They are thinkers eager to question assumptions, diplomats skilled at communication with those who are suffering and vulnerable, and jugglers always balancing their many responsibilities.

CONCLUSION: A NEW OUTLOOK

What do these trends mean for government entities (such as the National Institutes of Health [NIH] in the United States) in terms of the return on investment and the fulfillment of the overall goals of these programs? In short, we feel that the NIH should expand its view of how these programs return their investment. The value of training MD-PhDs is summed up as more than just clinical output or research productivity from those who stay on track to become pure physician-scientists in the academic sense.

We should consider how MD-PhDs contribute to education, communication in the public sphere, civil service, and broader social change. While generalization of expertise can be problematic in certain ways, combined MD-PhD training should lead those who complete it to believe that you can do anything as a physician-scientist. The training one receives as an MD-PhD is unique and thus can be used in many different ways, all of which can be defined as success.

31

Training a Diverse Physician-Scientist Workforce

Lashanda Skerritt

Lashanda Skerritt *is a fourth-year MD-PhD Candidate at McGill University. She is pursuing her PhD in family medicine and primary care. Her dissertation focuses on reproductive health care for women living with HIV. In 2016, she founded a mentorship program aimed at supporting high school students from underrepresented groups in medicine to explore careers in health care.*

INTRODUCTION

Increasing diversity in academic medicine has been a priority for many years. Despite marginal improvements, programs are still struggling with it. This chapter explains the under-discussed issue of diversity within the physician-scientist workforce, recognizing the feelings of marginalization that students from underrepresented groups may experience. The chapter aims to provide concrete advice for success as an MD-PhD student and an underrepresented minority.

The physician-scientist workforce has historically been a place of underrepresentation for groups who identify as women, Black, Indigenous, People of Colour LGBTQ+, and from low socioeconomic status. Some strides have been made. For instance, a generation ago, women made up a small proportion of MD and MD-PhD programs. Now, women are equally

> **WHAT YOU NEED TO KNOW**
>
> - Some MD-PhD programs have a diversity issue that combines many of the factors that contribute to underrepresentation in medicine and graduate studies.
> - Underrepresented minorities should build effective mentorship relationships with a diversity of mentors.
> - Don't overlook the importance of sponsors. Sponsors use their organizational capital and credibility to create opportunities to help you advance in your career.
> - Maintaining relationships outside of medicine and academia can help to combat feelings of isolation as a minority.
> - Take advantage of resources created to provide equitable support for minorities.

represented or account for more than half of MD-only and MD-PhD training programs in the United States and Canada. However, women are underrepresented among MD-PhD grant holders and in senior academic positions. Compared to men, women MD-PhDs are less likely to pursue and advance in careers in academic medicine after completing their training. The disparity is even greater in leadership positions. In essence, gender discrepancy in the physician-scientist workforce is not an issue of recruitment but rather of retention.

On the other hand, although retention is an issue in the MD-PhD pathway for Black, Indigenous and People of Colour students, so is recruitment. These students are severely underrepresented among MD-PhD program matriculants. Moreover, diversity and inclusivity issues have been reported among LGBTQ+ medical students. Fear of discrimination prevents non-cis-gender students from disclosing their gender identity. Lack of support in training programs also contributes to the underrepresentation of students with disabilities, including hearing, vision, cognitive, mobility, and independence impairments. Supporting a diverse population of MD-PhD trainees is essential to establishing a diverse, productive, and innovative workforce of physician-scientists.

This chapter positions the topic of diversity within the context of physician-scientist training, written with underrepresented minorities in mind. If you identify as an underrepresented minority and are considering, beginning, or pursuing MD-PhD training, this chapter describes the current landscape among MD-PhD trainees and physician-scientists, and touches on some of the reasons for underrepresentation. I want to emphasize that as a minority, it is not your responsibility to fix diversity issues, although at times you may be asked to do so (more on that later). Your responsibility as an MD-PhD trainee is to get the best education possible to help you succeed in your career. This chapter is meant to equip you with information and specific strategies to navigate the challenging physician-scientist landscape as an underrepresented minority. Diversity issues are complex, and for the sake of confining this topic to one chapter, the complexity is not explored in-depth but instead is briefly described to situate specific considerations and strategies to succeed as a minority. Drawing on my own experiences, I describe how to build and leverage relationships with mentors, sponsors, support networks, and financial resources as a minority MD-PhD trainee.

WHO IS REPRESENTED AMONG MD-PhD TRAINEES?

Diversity has become an important focus in many sectors, including government, industry, and academia. Diverse teams and workplaces are more productive and innovative, with deep cross-cultural connections yielding greater creativity. This is seen among entrepreneurs, designers, academic researchers, health care workers, and students. There is also evidence suggesting that disparities in health care workforce diversity are detrimental to patient care. A health care workforce that reflects the diversity of the patient population is one of the many approaches needed to improve health inequities. In response, medical schools have implemented efforts to increase diversity in the physician-scientist pipeline.

Addressing the diversity issues in the physician-scientist workforce requires recognition of the historical and social role of racism, sexism, and classism. In 1954, the US Supreme Court case *Brown v. Board of Education of Topeka* concluded with a unanimous ruling against the racial segregation of public schools. In 1964, the Civil Rights Act led to the desegregation and integration of institutions of higher education throughout the United States. Despite these landmark legal decisions that were meant to make higher education accessible to Black students in the United States, We still observe racial inequities in access to education. Since the inception of MD-PhD programs in the United States, the proportion of graduates who identify as Black is strikingly lower than US population demographics. The realities of underrepresentation are similar for many other groups, including Indigenous and Latinx MD-PhDs. Today, increasing participation of minorities (ethnic, gender, sexual orientation, and ability) has become an important initiative for many agencies that fund MD-PhD training programs. Despite the recognized importance of building a diverse workforce of physician-scientists, trainee diversity still lags behind that of medical schools, which also face their own diversity issues.

In 2018, half of MD-PhD matriculants across the United States identified as white and a quarter identified as Asian. Indigenous, Black, and Latinx students are strikingly underrepresented when compared to national racial/ethnicity demographics. Moreover, gender differences are seen among program graduates; women are dropping out of MD-PhD programs at higher rates compared to men.

Data on the racial/ethnic composition of Canadian MD-PhD trainees are not readily available; however, data from 2017 indicate that the female students account for around 40% of MD-PhD trainees compared to almost 60% of MD-only trainees.

UNDERSTANDING THE LEAKY PIPELINE

On the path toward successful academic careers as physician-scientists, many minorities are lost due to systemic issues. The loss of minorities along the physician-scientist pipeline combines diversity issues within medicine and graduate training programs. As a minority trying to navigate this training environment, remember that it is not your job to fix these systemic issues. Your job is to focus on your training and education so that you can achieve your career goals. To do this, however, requires resilience and strategic thinking. While programs work to address the larger systemic issues, it helps for you to understand the reasons for underrepresentation so that you can develop strategies to make it to the end of the pipeline.

The leaky pipeline in medicine

The leaky pipeline of diverse physician-scientists combines two issues: the lack of diversity among medical students and physicians, and the issues of underrepresentation among PhD students. Underrepresentation remains an issue in medical education despite efforts that have been made to increase diversity. In 2009, the Liaison Committee on Medical Education (LCME) introduced formal accreditation guidelines that required medical schools to develop programs or partnerships designed to "make admission to medical education more accessible to potential applicants of diverse backgrounds." Studies examining racial demographics among medical undergraduates, graduates, and faculty have reported modest improvements since the LCME guidelines were established. However, when proportions are adjusted for changes in US population demographics, this trend toward increased representation is no longer significant. Minorities are still underrepresented in the pool of applicants and matriculants. Poor investment in public education and disparities in educational resource allocation have been cited as societal contributors to lack of diversity in the medical school pipeline.

The leaky pipeline in academia

The situation is similar among doctoral students. Underrepresentation has been attributed to social factors, including the cost of attending college, pre-college preparation, lack of opportunity, and lack of mentorship and guidance. College graduation rates are lower among women and underrepresented minorities in the fields of science, technology, engineering, and math (STEM). Representation among students pursuing bachelor's degrees in STEM has improved, but this improvement is not seen among students pursuing master's and doctoral degrees.

For instance, White non-Hispanic males and females accounted for the largest percentage of graduate students in neuroscience programs, while Indigenous males and females represented fewer than 1% of graduate students. A history of colonialization, including a denial of the validity of Indigenous knowledge within educational institutions and a lack of education about the consequences of colonialization, encourages the persistence of discrimination against Indigenous students in higher education.

In general, the proportion of underrepresented minorities in graduate programs in STEM has not changed, despite efforts made by the National Science Foundation, the National Institutes of Health (NIH), and college and university faculty to increase minority enrollment, retention, and graduation. Although the proportion of Black PhD graduates has increased modestly over the past decade, there are still many fields (mostly within STEM) where each year not a single doctoral degree was awarded to a Black person throughout the United States. The issue of cost has been cited as a barrier for many Black students. Black college students borrow at higher rates than any other racial group, and they are more likely to default on those loans. Adding 8 years of training, the typical time it takes to complete the MD-PhD, after an undergraduate degree can be daunting. Moreover, the retention of underrepresented minority students along the pathway from high school to PhD further decreases during postdoctoral training and in the early-career stages for an independent researcher.

The doubly leaky physician-scientist pipeline

Matriculation in and graduation from an MD-PhD program combine many of these obstacles. Although the cost of training is significantly higher in the United States, financial disincentives to pursuing a career as a physician-scientist have been observed in Canada as well. The prolonged training with very little income as a student is a significant disincentive for prospective MD-PhD students. Although most programs provide stipends that cover tuition and basic living expenses, meaning that MD-PhD students graduate with less debt than their MD-only classmates, there is still a perception of difficulty in obtaining funding in the future and the disincentive of lower salaries and delayed earnings.

To accommodate their research and academic work, physician-scientists often conduct less clinical work than their physician-only colleagues. This often means physician-scientists have lower earnings than their colleagues in the same medical specialty. Income and delayed earnings may be a major motivator for a variety of circumstances, including paying off student loans and supporting one's family. For those who are more focused on maximizing earnings, a career as a physician-scientist is less appealing. This may contribute to the lower number of applicants from low-income households pursuing this career path. It is important to note, however, that although physician-scientists may have lower earnings in the short- and long-term compared to their physician-only colleagues, physician-scientists generally report feeling well-compensated.

WHY SO MANY WOMEN LEAVE ACADEMIC MEDICINE

Women who complete their MD-PhD training are less likely to pursue careers in academic medicine (teaching, seeing patients, conducting research) compared to graduates who identify as men. For women MD-PhDs who do go on to pursue academic medicine, the percentage who advance drops at each step of the pathway from graduate to assistant professor to associate professor to full professor.

Women experience a unique combination of barriers that hinder their careers in academia. First, women are less likely to be promoted to higher posts in academia. The underrepresentation of women on promotion committees has been cited as one reason for the declining representation of women at the levels of associate and full professor. Moreover, women are less likely to cite their own publications and negotiate for career advancement, two factors that impact promotion. Second, gender bias and social norms contribute to the gendered discrepancies in teaching evaluations by students. Women professors are more likely to be called emotional and unfair by students and less likely to be called experts. Gender biases have also been observed in peer-review evaluations for research grants and career awards, where women principal investigators were assessed less favorably than their counterparts who were men. This illustrates the gender biases in academic medicine that hinder career advancement for women physician-scientists.

Physician-scientists are constantly challenged with the task of not only establishing but also integrating their physician and researcher identities. Physician-scientists invest a lot of time cultivating a meaningful and fulfilling career. Many physician-scientists also try to maintain satisfying personal lives. For many, this includes starting and/or caring for their families. For many women, their MD-PhD training occupies most of their reproductive years. Family planning has not been shown to directly affect women's decisions to pursue MD-PhD training, but there is evidence from other sectors, including business, that indicates it may play into women's career decision making.

Women who chose to undertake MD-PhD training do so because they are ambitious. They undertake a challenging career path and perhaps are not initially thinking about starting a family. Over time, having children may ascend the list of priorities for many women. A woman may decide that pursuing an MD over an MD-PhD fits better with her plans to start a family and raise children, or that not pursuing an MD-PhD may fit better with her caregiving responsibilities. This is not a fault of women, but rather the consequence of work and social settings that are not supportive of all the roles and responsibilities women are tasked with. Society still places most caregiving responsibilities on women, meaning women may spend less time pursuing their professional goals because of the responsibilities of childcare, elder care, etc. Chapter 29 described in greater detail specific considerations for women physician-scientists. For women considering whether pursuing an MD-PhD conflicts with plans to start and raise their families, it is important to recognize that many women with children have successful careers as physician-scientists. It is possible to simultaneously find fulfillment in your career and family life as a woman physician-scientist.

UNDERREPRESENTATION AMONG FACULTY

Obstacles to grant success

Like discrepancies in research funding competitions between men and women scientists, discrepancies in research funding between Black and White researchers have also been observed.

Black scientists are less likely to apply for National Institutes of Health (NIH) R01 research grants. An R01 is the most common research project grant, which provides support to a principal investigator for several years, allowing them time (typically 3–5 years) and financial resources to conduct research, publish, and secure additional funding for their future research. To receive this grant, an independent investigator must submit an application, which is then reviewed by a committee of experts in the subject matter. Funding is awarded to the applications that the committee deems the most meritorious. Racial disparities were found in which grants were reviewed and which were funded. As grants are crucial to promotion and success in academic medicine, this creates a huge barrier for Black researchers to advance in academic medicine.

Discrimination in the workplace

Women and underrepresented minorities have described their academic work environment as unwelcoming, hostile, and discriminatory. Lack of mentorship, sponsorship, and barriers to promotion have all been cited as reasons for avoiding or leaving academic medicine. Even the portraiture within these institutions has been described as an obvious illustration of racism, sexism, and elitism. Often, medical schools hang portraits of former deans or faculty. In the majority of cases, all or most of these are portraits of White men. This lack of representation contradicts the messages of diversity and inclusivity that programs wish to convey. Some academic medical centers have begun to remove portraits in recognition of their conflicting message about diversity, but portraiture is just one example of why minorities might feel unwelcome.

Underrepresented minorities have decried the lack of role models and challenges identifying mentors and sponsors to help them navigate and advance in their careers. (Advice for minorities on leveraging mentorship and sponsorship is provider later in this chapter.) Representation within faculty has been found to be strongly associated with diversity among medical students. In other words, minorities are more likely to study medicine in programs where they see minority faculty represented.

The minority tax

Underrepresentation among faculty has also been attributed to the "minority tax." The minority tax is a concept that refers to the additional responsibilities placed on minority faculty to help their institutions with diversity, equity, and inclusiveness efforts. Faculty from underrepresented minorities are often expected to mentor students from underrepresented groups, chair diversity and inclusivity committees, and represent the voices of other minorities. Their participation in initiatives aimed at increasing diversity are rarely recognized or compensated. I have experienced this firsthand. My interest in diversity and equity issues within medicine led me to join an equity and inclusivity committee at my medical school. The experience was very enriching, bringing together health professions faculty, students, and committee members to find solutions to underrepresentation in health professions programs. My membership on this committee led to me being expected or asked to participate in many other equity and diversity initiatives at my medical school. Although I wanted to be involved in these initiatives, I also found it overwhelming to try to balance these activities on top of my medical school classes, research, and other activities.

As minority faculty often represent a small sample within their institutions, feeling overburdened is a common experience. On top of the additional expectations placed on minority faculty, they also experience feelings of isolation due to the perception of being the only minority in their research or clinical settings. Despite research reporting that diverse perspectives enrich collaboration and outcomes, which benefits the institution and health care system, negative stereotyping about minority faculty in academic medicine is still documented. Minority faculty are more likely to be viewed as less educated and lacking research skills. Moreover, experiences of discrimination have been cited as reasons why some minority faculty feel that they have to constantly prove their worth and abilities more than their colleagues. All of these factors and the resilience needed to manage them are, understandably, taxing for underrepresented minorities.

STRATEGIES FOR NAVIGATING MD-PhD TRAINING AS AN UNDERREPRESENTED MINORITY

A diverse physician-scientist workforce is needed to address the complex needs of a diverse patient population. The existing lack of diversity and obstacles faced by minorities calls for concerted efforts to increase participation of those from different ethnicities, socioeconomic status, gender identity, sexual orientation, and personal experiences. Strategies for underrepresented minorities to succeed in this environment include recognizing the importance of mentorship and sponsorship, finding a community where you feel valued, and having financial support throughout your training.

MAKE YOUR RELATIONSHIPS WITH MENTORS WORK FOR YOU

Build a diverse mentorship network

Longitudinal mentorship plays an important role throughout training and even as an established physician-scientist. Effective mentorship can help to address barriers to physician-scientist success. Having functional mentorship relationships is also associated with greater career satisfaction. Mentors do not necessarily need to have the same background or life experiences, but they do need to be compassionate and understanding of the unique struggles that certain groups face. Mentors can be a helpful resource when applying to programs and providing guidance to help you achieve your training and career goals.

Even after formal training has ended, mentors can help address other issues, such as the racial and gender gap in acquiring research funding, by providing feedback on grant applications or being co-applicants on a grant. Chapter 10 provided strategies to go about identifying an academic mentor who will supervise your research and development throughout your doctoral studies. Drawing on the advice and experience of a diversity of mentors, however, can be a strategy to maximize the benefits of mentorship.

Finding a mentor can sometimes be challenging. The label "mentor" puts pressure on both the mentee and the mentor to develop a specific type of relationship. The relationship itself is more important than the label. It is not always the best approach to ask people in senior positions to mentor you. These relationships often develop organically as you ask questions and share obstacles and successes with those more advanced in their careers. However, access to mentors is not always equitable, justifying the need for formal mentorship programs to help those who may not be as well-connected in their field.

Foster relationships that are positive for you and your mentors

You want the experience of mentoring you to be a positive one for your mentor. One approach that can be taken to establish the relationship is to have a positive, thought-out approach in all of your interactions with a potential mentor. Be prepared for each meeting with specific problems or questions you wish to discuss. These questions are opportunities to seek advice from a potential mentor and should not be easily answered with a Google search. You want to demonstrate that you value the time spent with a mentor and want to make the most of it. Some of the questions I've approached my mentors with have included whether it was worthwhile to sit on another diversity/equity/inclusivity committee or participate in another diversity initiative. Mentors can offer valuable advice on when to say no.

Seek mentors with identities and experiences different from your own

Mentoring is an essential component of career development. Mentor-mentee relationships often form between people with similar backgrounds and interests. For example, Senior men are more likely to mentor young men who remind them of themselves. Since there is a shortage of women in leadership roles, young women need to expand their pool of mentors to include men. Until complete gender equity is achieved, women still require mentorship and sponsorship from leaders to ascend in their careers, and leaders at present are overwhelmingly men. Unfortunately, men in various sectors have begun to express hesitation about mentoring young female colleagues in the wake of #MeToo, adding another barrier to mentorship for women.

As a woman physician-scientist trainee, you should approach men in leadership as potential mentors. To address any fear of one-on-one meetings being misconstrued, you can offer to meet in public spaces. This might mean that the first few meetings happen over coffee in the hospital cafeteria. As you get to know each other more, the settings might change, but use your judgment to decide on meeting spaces where you and your mentor will feel comfortable.

Take advantage of mentorship programs

Some MD-PhD programs may have established formal mentorship programs to provide coaching and teaching circles so that mentors can learn from each other and share successes and challenges. While some may argue that mentor-mentee relationships are best left to develop organically, not everyone has the same opportunities to connect with the right people in the right settings to foster such connections. Mentoring opportunities should be available equitably. Although not everyone will need or benefit from a formal mentorship program, its existence may create opportunities for those with more barriers to establishing a relationship with a mentor. Formal mentorship programs are also great because they often provide education and guidelines for mentors on issues such as unconscious bias or fears that some men might have regarding mentoring women after #MeToo. If these exist in your institution, take advantage of the opportunities and resources they provide.

Pipeline programs for underrepresented minorities have been established to help students become competitive applicants, successful MD-PhD students, and future researchers in academic medicine. These types of programs provide students with much-needed exposure to careers as physician-scientists, but the support often ends when participation in the program ends. Longitudinal mentorship is harder to establish but incredibly important to support your success. After participating in these types of programs, reach out to the program directors or researchers that you meet. Find ways to stay in touch, such as volunteering in their lab or at research days or conferences.

MOVE BEYOND MENTORSHIP AND LEVERAGE SPONSORSHIP

Your network is a group of people whom you can go to for advice, support, and perspective. This network should include both mentors and sponsors. Over the course of my academic career, I have built my network of teachers, professors, supervisors, colleagues, and peers, many of whom have acted as my sponsors, advocating for me at different stages of my training.

A sponsor is someone in a position of power or influence who can leverage their position to actively advocate for you publicly and behind closed doors. Sponsorship is important for securing critical roles and responsibilities that help to advance your career as a physician-scientist. This might mean recommending you for a teaching or guest-lecturing position, suggesting you as an author for a book chapter, or putting in a good word formally (letter of recommendation) or informally to help you secure a postdoc position. Sponsors use their organizational capital to advocate for the investment of time, resources, and expertise to support your development. Sponsorship is particularly important for women, who, evidence shows, are over-mentored and under-sponsored. The role of a sponsor differs from a mentor in that a mentor will help you to develop your skills and abilities, guiding you on which skills to develop and how. A sponsor, on the other hand, knows your skills and abilities, identifies your potential, and finds opportunities to champion you.

When I was searching for a lab and supervisor for my doctoral research, I asked my previous supervisor for advice about how to identify a good supervisor. She drew on her own experiences during her PhD and postdoc, offering guidance on things that I had not considered. She even helped to connect me with a potential supervisor whom she knew from her postdoc. She recommended that I use her name and position to help bolster my credibility. In an environment such as academia where bias is rampant, having someone in a position of power speak about you favorably can make a huge difference. Similarly, my peers have also been my sponsors, helping me to identify opportunities, including teaching positions, conferences, collaborations, and scholarships.

NURTURE YOUR SUPPORT NETWORK WITHIN AND BEYOND MEDICINE AND ACADEMIA

Networking is part of building your community, and successful networks will look quite different for different people and different groups of people, including across race and gender. Physician-scientists from underrepresented groups have found communities through social media. #Diversedoubledocs is a social media hashtag that was created by the American Physician Scientists Association to highlight diversity. Physician-scientist trainees from across North America use this hashtag to tweet about their unique experiences, share resources, answer questions from prospective students, and encourage each other. Engaging in these discussions virtually can also help to foster feelings of belonging, especially if you feel alone within your home institution.

Research has shown that the networks of successful men and women have one crucial difference. Successful women have a network that includes a close inner circle of women. A network with this inner circle of women helps to advance a woman's career by pointing out gender-related tacit information. This may include avoiding a work environment with a culture of gender bias or women drawing on their own networks to identify or create opportunities for other women. I think of my close network of amazing women PhD students and postdocs who have helped me navigate some of the nuanced experiences of academic research as a woman. This has even included pointing out instances where I have written about my accomplishments humbly in scholarship applications, a common practice for many women who are taught to be humble from an early age.

Your network also includes your family and friends. Having this support outside of your professional network helps to keep things in perspective. Of course, there may be some annoyances. At every family function, I find myself re-explaining the timeline of my training program. My family members regularly ask me how much longer I will be in school, and whether I am in medical school or graduate school, but the questions emerge because this is all new to them. I will be the first in my family to earn an MD and the first in my immediate family to finish graduate school. It requires patience to field these questions, but I've decided that keeping my family up-to-date about my progress is worth the effort.

Knowing that I have a group of people who care about me and want to see me succeed motivates me and also makes me accountable. I feel that they are just as invested in my success as I am, and that helps me to keep going. Given the independent nature of the PhD, isolation is commonly felt by most graduate students at some point in their training. Qualitative research has revealed that students from underrepresented minorities are even more sensitive to that experience. Having a community of support is essential for any physician-scientist to be successful and even more so for minorities.

RESEARCH FINANCIAL RESOURCES AND SUPPORT AVAILABLE TO YOU DURING YOUR TRAINING

The prospect of delayed earning may be a disincentive for some considering MD-PhD training. Most programs, however, provide financial support throughout your studies. MD-PhD students graduate with less debt on average compared to their MD-only colleagues. In addition, many scholarship opportunities are available during the graduate portion of the training program to provide financial assistance. With the proper resources and support, the cost of completing an MD-PhD can be managed and mitigated. For trainees in American programs, it is useful to familiarize yourself with funding opportunities developed specifically to provide equitable financial support for minorities. The NIH Research Supplements to Promote Diversity in Health-Related Research are an example.

CONCLUSION

Progress on diversity issues in MD-PhD programs has been made, but inequities in support and opportunities still exist, preventing some people in minority groups from embarking on and succeeding in a career as a physician-scientist. Women and underrepresented minorities experience greater barriers to career success. Changes are needed at the institutional and societal levels to ensure equal opportunities for everyone. It is not the role of minorities to fix these larger structural issues. In the current climate, women and underrepresented minorities can position themselves for greater success by pursuing their career ambitions at full speed, identifying mentors and sponsors to help them achieve their career goals, building a community of support that includes peers, family, and friends, and, finally, leveraging existing resources to financially support their MD-PhD journey.

32

Closing Remarks

Staying on the Physician-Scientist Path
Written by Dr. Andrea L. Cox

We hope that The Essential MD-PhD Guide has helped you to determine if the physician-scientist path is right for you or to navigate the physician-scientist path if you have already chosen this wonderful career. Clinical medicine and research have many synergies that permit the well-trained physician-scientist to succeed in both arenas.

MD-PhD programs take advantage of synergies in training that reduce the time to degree compared to earning both degrees separately and permit students to focus on clinical and research excellence simultaneously. Both MD-PhD programs and Physician-Scientist Training Programs (PSTPs) allow physician-scientists in training to come together to share support, encouragement, and advice with like-minded individuals. We recommend that you seek out events between PSTPs and MD-PhD programs and physician-scientist meetings outside your institution to extend the network of people with common goals and interests beyond your own program.

Role models and advisors who encourage people of all races, ethnic groups, and genders to pursue scientific and medical excellence will be key for continuing on this path. Engage successful mentors willing to hold regular and open discussions with you about their physician-scientist careers. If you are a member of a group underrepresented among physician-scientists, you may need to seek mentoring from supportive sources outside your own gender, ethnic, or racial group until the physician-scientist work force is more representative of the general population. Having mentors from different backgrounds can actually benefit all trainees and learning from people with diverse perspectives is critical to forming and maintaining a supportive mentoring network. At later stages, connecting with senior mentors who have the financial capacity to support researchers can be key because junior faculty awards often lack sufficient research funds to perform meaningful research and sharing expensive equipment is beneficial. A factor to consider in choosing where to pursue the physician-scientist career is workplace culture. Staying up to date with advances in patient care and research is greatly facilitated by a workplace culture that inspires open collaboration and the free exchange of knowledge and resources.

On the personal side, if you are choosing a partner, finding a supportive partner is no less important. Having a life partner who understands and values your career, who shares the workload at home, and who celebrates your success makes life so much easier and fun than a partner who is not highly supportive. Do not try to do everything yourself. Paying professionals to perform household tasks you don't enjoy and are not any better suited to than others can free up time for work responsibilities and much needed down time, exercise, and recreation.

In addition to the pleasure of caring for patients, physician-scientists have the opportunity to do research that changes the standard of care for many more patients than they could treat in a lifetime. Success is far more likely to occur if you choose a field of medicine and research about which you are intensely passionate – go with your heart rather than what you think is in vogue or an area of societal need that is not of great interest to you. In sum, focus on quality of life and support strategies that have proven successful in encouraging talented people to thrive on the physician-scientist path and you too will experience the joys of research with the potential to transform the care of patients. We hope you find this career as gratifying, exciting, and fulfilling as we have.

Mark J. Eisenberg, MD MPH
Director, MD PhD ProgramDirector,
Cardiovascular Health Services Research
ProgramMcGill UniversityMontréal,
Quebec

Andrea L. Cox, MD PhD
Director, MD PhD Program
Johns Hopkins University
Baltimore, Maryland

Index

www.ingramcontent.com/pod-product-compliance
Lightning Source LLC
Chambersburg PA
CBHW082110220326
41598CB00066BA/6057